Occupational Medicine

STATE OF THE ART REVIEWS

Tuberculosis in the Workplace

Guest Editor:

Steven B. Markowitz, MD
Division of Environmental and Occupational Medicine
Department of Community Medicine
Mount Sinai School of Medicine
New York, New York

Volume 9/Number 4 October–December 1994
HANLEY & BELFUS, INC. Philadelphia

Publisher: HANLEY & BELFUS, INC.
210 South 13th Street
Philadelphia, PA 19107
(215) 546-4995
Fax (215) 790-9330

OCCUPATIONAL MEDICINE: State of the Art Reviews is included in *Index Medicus, MEDLINE, BioSciences Information Service, Current Contents* and *ISI/BIOMED.*

OCCUPATIONAL MEDICINE: State of the Art Reviews **(ISSN 0885-114X)**
October–December 1994 **Volume 9, Number 4** **(ISBN 1-56053-175-4)**

OCCUPATIONAL MEDICINE: State of the Art Reviews is published quarterly by Hanley & Belfus, Inc., 210 South 13th Street, Philadelphia, Pennsylvania 19107. Second-class postage paid at Philadelphia, PA and at additional mailing offices.

POSTMASTER: Send address changes to OCCUPATIONAL MEDICINE: State of the Art Reviews, Hanley & Belfus, Inc., 210 South 13th Street, Philadelphia, PA 19107.

The 1994 subscription price is $82.00 per year U.S., $92.00 outside U.S. (add $40.00 for air mail).

Occupational Medicine: State of the Art Reviews
Vol. 9, No. 4, October–December 1994

TUBERCULOSIS IN THE WORKPLACE
Steven B. Markowitz, MD, Editor

CONTENTS

In this comprehensive review, the authors describe various types of respirators and the major issues in their application to TB control, including the degree of protection they offer and cost. Recent recommendations regarding the use of respiratory protective devices also are discussed.

It was not until several health care unions petitioned OSHA for a bloodborne pathogen standard in 1986 that OSHA began to play a major role in regulating the health care industry. The authors examine the Service Employees International Union's current effort to urge OSHA to develop a standard to protect workers from occupational exposure to TB. They also cover ramifications of the CDC's revised guidelines for preventing the transmission of TB in health care settings.

The authors argue that the classic hierarchy of industrial hygiene controls may be successfully used to control TB. Various elements of hygiene control programs reviewed here include TB exposure control programs, identification and isolation of patients, respiratory isolation, local source capture ventilation, laboratory procedures, employee surveillance programs, reporting of occupational illnesses, labeling requirements, and respiratory protection.

After outlining the basics of workplace training programs regarding tuberculosis, the authors describe the experiences of Hunter College, the New York Committee for Occupational Safety and Health, and the New York State Public Employees Federation in developing TB education programs. A resource guide lists agencies and organizations that can be contacted for information on tuberculosis control, educational programs, and training curricula.

This detailed discussion of medical surveillance techniques addresses such issues as the administration and interpretation of the tuberculin skin test, the importance of BCG vaccine, preventive therapy with isoniazid, the identification of groups at high risk for TB, multidrug-resistant tuberculosis, and regulatory requirements for PPD testing, including CDC guidelines.

CONTRIBUTORS

Edward Anselm, MD
Director, Employee Health Services, Empire Blue Cross and Blue Shield, New York, New York

Christopher C. Coffey, MS
Research Chemist, Division of Safety Research, National Institute for Occupational Safety and Health, Morgantown, West Virginia

Jamie Cohen, BS
Assistant Director, Health and Safety Department, Service Employees International Union, Washington, DC

Ronald P. DePersis, BA
Research Scientist II—Industrial Hygiene, New York State Department of Health, Bureau of Occupational Health, Albany, New York

Charles P. Felton, MD
Clinical Professor of Medicine, Department of Medicine, Columbia University College of Physicians and Surgeons, New York, New York

Jean G. Ford, MD
Assistant Professor of Medicine, Department of Medicine, Columbia University College of Physicians and Surgeons, New York, New York

N.A. Gillen, BS
United States Department of Labor, Occupational Safety and Health Administration, New York, New York

Lee Hathon, PE, MSPH
Salt Lake City, Utah

Thomas K. Hodous, MD
Chief, Science and Policy Coordination, Division of Safety Research, National Institute for Occupational Safety and Health, and Adjunct Professor, Department of Medicine, West Virginia University School of Medicine, Morgantown, West Virginia

Pamela Kellner, RN, MPH
New York City Department of Health, New York, New York

Laura Kenny, MPH
Assistant Director, Health and Safety Department, Service Employees International Union, New York, New York

Susan Klitzman, DrPH
New York City Department of Health, New York, New York

Matthew A. London, MS
Industrial Hygienist, New York State Department of Health, Albany, New York

Steven B. Markowitz, MD
Associate Professor, Division of Environmental and Occupational Medicine, Department of Community Medicine, Mount Sinai School of Medicine, New York, New York

Melissa A. McDiarmid, MD, MPH
Director, Office of Occupational Medicine, United States Department of Labor, Occupational Safety and Health Administration, Washington, DC

James Melius, MD, DrPH
Director, Division of Occupational Health and Environmental Epidemiology, New York State Department of Health, Albany, New York

Jacqueline M. Moline, MD, MSc
Instructor, Department of Community Medicine, Mount Sinai School of Medicine, New York, New York

Deborah A. Nagin, MPH
Research Scientist—Industrial Hygiene, New York State Department of Health, Environmental and Occupational Health, New York, New York

Nicholas Pavelchak
Research Scientist—Industrial Hygiene, New York State Department of Health, Bureau of Occupational Health, Albany, New York

David N. Rose, MD
Associate Professor, Departments of Community Medicine and Medicine, Mount Sinai School of Medicine, New York, New York

Jonathan D. Rosen, BS
Director, Occupational Health and Safety Department, New York State Public Employees Federation, AFL-CIO, Albany, New York

Lisa H. Watson, MPH
Associate Director, New York Committee for Occupational Safety and Health, New York, New York

1994 ISSUES

Occupational Skin Disease
Edited by James R. Nethercott, MD
University of Maryland
Baltimore, Maryland

Occupational Safety and Health Training
Edited by Michael J. Colligan, PhD
National Institute for Occupational Safety and Health
Cincinnati, Ohio

Reproductive Hazards
Edited by Ellen B. Gold, PhD,
B. L. Lasley, PhD, and
Marc B. Schenker, MD, MPH
University of California
Davis, California

Tuberculosis in the Workplace
Edited by Steven Markowitz, MD
Mount Sinai School of Medicine
New York, New York

1993 ISSUES

The Mining Industry
Edited by Daniel E. Banks, MD
West Virginia University
Morgantown, West Virginia

De Novo Toxicants
Edited by Dennis J. Shusterman, MD, MPH
California EPA, Berkeley, California
and Jack E. Peterson, PhD, CIH
Alpine, California

Spirometry
Edited by Ellen A. Eisen, ScD
University of Massachusetts
Lowell, Massachusetts

Women Workers
Edited Dana M. Headapohl, MD
St. Patrick's Hospital
Missoula, Montana

1992 ISSUES

Back School Programs
Edited by Lynne A. White
Director, Practice Management Resources
San Francisco, California

Occupational Lung Disease
Edited by William S. Beckett, MD
Yale University School of Medicine
New Haven, Connecticut
and Rebecca Bascom, MD
University of Maryland School of Medicine
Baltimore, Maryland

Unusual Occupational Diseases
Edited by Dennis J. Shusterman, MD, MPH
Berkeley, California
and Paul D. Blanc, MD, MSPH
University of California, San Francisco
San Francisco, California

Ergonomics
Edited by J. Steven Moore, MD
Medical College of Wisconsin
and Arun Garg, PhD
University of Wisconsin–Milwaukee
Milwaukee, Wisconsin

Ordering Information:
Subscriptions for full year and single issues are available from the publisher—
Hanley & Belfus, Inc., 210 South 13th Street, Philadelphia, PA 19107.
Telephone (215) 546-7293; (800) 962-1892. Fax (215) 790-9330.

PUBLISHED ISSUES

(available from the publisher)

Vol 2/No 2 Apr.–June 1987	**Occupational Pulmonary Disease** Edited by Linda Rosenstock, MD, MPH
Vol 2/No 4 Oct.–Dec. 1987	**Workers with Multiple Chemical Sensitivities** Edited by Mark R. Cullen, MD
Vol 3/No 2 Apr.–June 1988	**Worker Fitness and Risk Evaluations** Edited by Jay S. Himmelstein, MD, MPH and Glenn S. Pransky, MD, MPH
Vol 3/No 3 July–Sept. 1988	**The Petroleum Industry** Edited by Neill K. Weaver, MD
Vol 3/No 4 Oct.–Dec. 1988	**Psychiatric Injury in the Workplace** Edited by Robert C. Larsen, MD, and Jean S. Felton, MD
Vol 4/No 1 Jan.–Mar. 1989	**The Management Perspective** Edited by L. Fleming Fallon, Jr., MD, MPH, MBA, O.B. Dickerson, MD, MPH, and Paul W. Brandt-Rauf, ScD, MD, DrPH
Vol 4/No 2 Apr.–June 1989	**Alcoholism and Chemical Dependency** Edited by Curtis Wright, MD, MPH
Vol 4/No 4 Oct.–Dec. 1989	**Problem Buildings** Edited by James E. Cone, MD, MPH and Michael Hodgson, MD, MPH
Vol 5/No 1 Jan.–Mar. 1990	**Hazardous Waste Workers** Edited by Michael Gochfeld, MD, PhD and Elissa Ann Favata, MD
Vol 5/No 2 Apr.–June 1990	**Shiftwork** Edited by Allene J. Scott, MD, MPH
Vol 5/No 3 July–Sept. 1990	**Medical Surveillance in the Workplace** Edited by David Rempel, MD, MPH
Vol 5/No 4 Oct.–Dec. 1990	**Worksite Health Promotion** Edited by Michael E. Scofield, PhD
Vol 6/No 1 Jan.–Mar. 1991	**Prevention of Pulmonary Disease in the Workplace** Edited by Philip Harber, MD, MPH and John R. Balmes, MD
Vol 6/No 2 Apr.–June 1991	**The Biotechnology Industry** Edited by Alan M. Ducatman, MD and Daniel F. Liberman, PhD
Vol 6/No 3 July–Sept. 1991	**Health Hazards of Farming** Edited by D. H. Cordes, MD, MPH and Dorothy Foster Rea, MS
Vol 6/No 4 Oct.–Dec. 1991	**The Nuclear Energy Industry** Edited by Gregg S. Wilkinson, PhD

PREFACE

Coming in the wake of the HIV epidemic, tuberculosis has stirred great concern among health care workers and those responsible for their occupational health care. To learn about the field of occupationally acquired tuberculosis, however, interested parties must consult journals from a wide variety of disciplines, obtain government documents, and track down reports that are unpublished or published with limited distribution. The goal of this volume is to synthesize scientific knowledge, public policy, and relevant opinion into a single, easily accessible source for health professionals and others who have interests in or responsibilities for workers at occupational risk of acquiring tuberculosis.

A clear consensus exists among all parties in the health care industry that primacy in attention and resource allocation must be given to the early identification and the appropriate and complete treatment of patients with tuberculosis. The occupational acquisition of tuberculosis will diminish as the incidence of tuberculosis in the general population decreases. There is much less of a consensus, however, about how much attention the occupational health aspects of the resurgence of tuberculosis deserve. This is demonstrated by the relative dearth of research on occupational tuberculosis and the small size of the budget devoted by federal agencies to investigating the risk of tuberculosis for workers and how to reduce this risk. We do not even have a simple and accurate count of the number of cases of occupational tuberculosis that occur each year in the United States.

Since the magnitude of the problem of occupational tuberculosis is not known, its impact cannot be used as the basis for arguing for increased resources and attention to the problem. Such an argument will clearly be ineffective when used to suggest that resources that otherwise might go for the identification and treatment of patients with active tuberculosis be used to protect workers. Rather, occupational tuberculosis demands attention, resources, and study, because workers have the legal (and moral) right to be protected from workplace hazards as mandated by the Occupational Health and Safety Act of 1970.

As expected in any topical area of science and policy, there is ongoing change in policies, guidelines and, to a lesser extent, scientific knowledge. The Occupational Health and Safety Administration is expected to issue a standard for airborne diseases, including tuberculosis, in 1995. By the date that this issue of the *State of the Art Reviews* is published, it is anticipated that the Centers for Disease Control and Prevention will have issued its final revised guidelines for the protection of health care workers from tuberculosis. The articles in this volume reflect the latest draft of the revised guidelines, which were issued in October 1993. The forthcoming final guidelines are not expected to be much different from the draft guidelines published in 1993, but the reader is advised to consult with the final guidelines in conjunction with reading the articles enclosed in this volume.

It is said that tuberculosis is a social disease with medical consequences. The same can be said for all occupational diseases.

STEVEN B. MARKOWITZ, MD
GUEST EDITOR

JEAN G. FORD, MD
CHARLES P. FELTON, MD

TUBERCULOSIS: PATHOGENESIS AND LABORATORY DIAGNOSIS

From the Department of Medicine
Columbia College of Physicians and Surgeons (JGF, CPF)
and
Division of Pulmonary Medicine
Harlem Hospital Center (JGF, CPF)
New York, New York

Reprint requests to:
Jean G. Ford, MD
Division of Pulmonary Medicine
Harlem Hospital Center
506 Malcolm X Boulevard
New York, NY 10037

The tuberculosis epidemic of the 1990s in the United States is occurring in a context that increases the likelihood of occupational spread compared to a mere two decades ago. The most important feature of this new epidemic is human immunodeficiency virus (HIV) infection, which causes rapid progression to tuberculosis disease in patients infected with *Mycobacterium tuberculosis* (Mtb).[55a] The challenge of preventing tuberculosis in the most severely affected communities is magnified by homelessness, substance abuse, and other psychiatric conditions, as well as a weak infrastructure for tuberculosis control.[10] Perhaps most ominous is the emergence of multidrug-resistant tuberculosis,[33] for which effective therapy takes longer and requires significantly more toxic and costly drugs.[34]

In this context, providers of services to patients with active tuberculosis are at increased risk of acquiring infection. In particular, workers in hospitals, jails and prisons, and other congregate living facilities are at increased risk of acquiring tuberculosis in the workplace through exposure to air infected with *M. tuberculosis*.[13 18]

On the other hand, emerging molecular biologic technologies hold the promise of more rapid diagnosis of disease,[28] more definitive epidemiologic linkage of cases of tuberculosis, and a greater appreciation of the extent of transmission of tuberculosis within communities[1,58] and institutions.[25] This could help to reduce markedly the period of infectiousness and nosocomial transmission of tuberculosis.

In this chapter, we review the pathogenesis of tuberculosis infection and discuss new methods for rapid detection of the disease.

PATHOGENESIS OF TUBERCULOSIS

The Mycobacterial Cell Wall

The genus *Mycobacterium* consists of more than 50 species that have the following common characteristics: (1) they are acid-fast, resisting decolorization by acid alcohol; (2) they are intracellular parasites and obligate aerobes; and (3) they have a slow rate of growth in vitro.[3,35]

Mycobacteria have a thick cell wall with a high lipid content, as well as proteins and peptides with strong tuberculin activity. The "backbone" of the mycobacterial cell wall, the peptidoglycan, is present in almost all bacteria. Lipopolysaccharide side chains that branch off this backbone are more specific, but they contain arabinogalactan, a polysaccharide also found in *Nocardia* and *Corynebacterium.* This polysaccharide is esterified at its distal end to mycolic acids, fatty acids that constitute the major part of the outer layer of the cell wall. In addition, mycolic acid residues are an important determinant of acid-fastness of mycobacteria. Since mycolic acids also occur in *Corynebacterium* and *Nocardia*, the lack of specificity of the acid-fast test is readily understandable.[3] Likewise, application of immunodiagnostic techniques that use arabinogalactan as antigen in serological tests is limited by cross-reactivity with antisera raised against *Corynebacteria*, *Nocardia*, and mycobacteria other than Mtb.

Pathogenesis of Tuberculous Infection

Transmission of Tuberculosis

The development of tuberculosis infection requires prolonged inhalation of air that is shared by a patient with active respiratory tuberculosis who has not been effectively treated. A patient who has infectious pulmonary or laryngeal tuberculosis contaminates ambient air by coughing or sneezing droplet nuclei containing *M. tuberculosis*. Once in the air, these droplet nuclei dry up rapidly, leaving the organism in the air. Unless they are removed by ventilation or bactericidal activity, these organisms may remain in the air for several hours.

Transmission of tuberculosis usually occurs in a variety of settings, where people at risk are likely to be exposed to infected air for prolonged periods, including hospitals, nursing homes, correctional facilities, homeless shelters, and the home environment.[6] Several factors determine the likelihood that a patient with active, infectious pulmonary tuberculosis will expose others to the organism. Factors related to the index case include the load of organisms released into the air, that is, whether the patient has cavitary or smear-positive disease, and the severity and duration of cough.[6] In addition, environmental factors such as poor ventilation and crowding increase the likelihood of exposure and consequent infection.[48,53]

Surveys of households of patients with tuberculosis indicate that 24–27% of those exposed to *M. tuberculosis* become infected.[6] Following initial exposure to the organism, the first line of host defense is nonimmunologic.[4,21] Some organisms are removed by filtration in the upper airway and impaction in large airways. Organisms that reach the ciliated epithelial surface of the conducting airways are moved upward toward the pharynx through the mucociliary escalator. They are then swallowed and killed by gastric acid,[4,21] or they may be expectorated.

Because *Mycobacterium tuberculosis* is a very small organism—1–4 μm long and 0.3–0.6 μm thick—it is readily inhaled deep into the lungs and into the alveoli.[3] The alveolar macrophage is the last line of defense against tuberculous infection. Alveolar macrophages migrate through the alveolus and subject foreign particles, including *M. tuberculosis*, to nonspecific phagocytosis.[4,21] Following fusion of phagosomes with lysosomes, organisms are killed by hydrolytic enzymes.[22]

Certain mycobacterial cell wall antigens,[44] particularly the sulfated acyl trehaloses, have been shown to prevent fusion of phagosomes with lysosomes in cultured macrophages infected with mycobacterium tuberculosis. This has led to the still-unproven hypothesis that these trehaloses are important determinants of mycobacterial virulence.[35,44]

Strain differences in phagocytosis by alveolar macrophages, and thus susceptibility to tuberculous infection, have been documented in guinea pigs.[60] This has been suggested as support for the hypothesis of differential racial susceptibility to tuberculosis infection on a genetic basis.[17] However, whether there is indeed differential susceptibility of alveolar macrophages to tuberculosis infection,[17] and to what extent this explains observed racial differences in rates of tuberculosis infection between African Americans and whites in the U.S., is the subject of substantial controversy.[29,30,38,61,62]

Since the alveolar macrophage is the last line of defense following exposure, inability of the alveolar macrophage to destroy the viable organism results in the onset of tuberculosis infection. This results in multiplication of tubercle bacilli within the macrophage, followed within 1 week by macrophage rupture and release of tubercle bacilli.[22] From the onset of infection until the development of specific cell-mediated immunity, a silent tuberculous bacillemia results in seeding of other lung sites and distant organs. Since killing of these organisms is incomplete, they may persist for years in a dormant state, but their containment depends on maintenance of an intact cell-mediated immune response.[40]

Chemotactic factors attract immature monocytes to this site, thereby initiating granuloma formation. Since these monocytes ingest the organisms but are incapable of destroying them, logarithmic growth of tubercle bacilli can be observed at this stage until the antigenic stimulus is sufficiently large to trigger delayed type hypersensitivity and cell-mediated immunity,[21] which usually occurs approximately 3 weeks following infection. At this point, monocytes are ruptured by cytotoxic lymphocytes, and macrophages are activated by previously sensitized lymphocytes to destroy ingested mycobacteria efficiently.[21] The result of this stage of the infection is immunologic control of primary infection through granuloma maturation. Thus, in the immunocompetent host, primary tuberculosis is usually subclinical, or it may cause mild disease, with self-limited symptoms.

Effects of HIV Infection on Tuberculous Infection and Progression

While tuberculosis infection often progresses to disease in people with the acquired immunodeficiency syndrome (AIDS),[55a] whether HIV-infected patients have an increased susceptibility to infection when exposed to *M. tuberculosis* remains a subject of debate.[18,47] On the other hand, the fairly common occurrence of exogenous reinfection of tuberculosis patients who are taking appropriate therapy is a sobering reminder of the central role of the immune system in preventing progression from tuberculosis infection to disease.[59]

The progressive immunodeficiency that characterizes HIV infection is mediated through the loss of CD_4 lymphocytes. CD_4 cells play a central role in the immune response. They provide specific help to CD_8 cytotoxic/suppressor lymphocytes, cells that appear to be important in the pathogenesis of tuberculosis. In addition, they produce cytokines and are central to the activation of macrophages against mycobacterial antigens. CD_4 lymphocytes also serve a helper function for cellular immunity. However, the latter does not appear to play a major role in the immunopathogenesis of tuberculosis. As increasing numbers of these cells are lost in the context of HIV infection, specific cellular derangements and alterations in cytokine production occur that are directly related to the rapid progression to disease in patients infected with HIV.[40]

Progressive Primary Tuberculosis

When host defenses are inadequate, tuberculosis infection may progress locally or systemically. In a host with an apparently normal immune system, an apical or subapical primary site may predispose to progressive primary tuberculosis.[47] While this early progression to disease has been known for decades to occur in a small percentage of patients, progressive primary tuberculosis is now most common in patients who have AIDS, are malnourished, receiving immunosuppressive therapy, or are otherwise immunologically compromised.[47]

Reactivation Tuberculosis

Reactivation tuberculosis may occur months to decades following recovery from the initial infection. Approximately 3–5% of people infected with Mtb will develop reactivation tuberculosis within the first year, and the risk declines progressively thereafter.[40] The risk of developing active disease is approximately 10% over a lifetime, given an intact immune system. However, HIV infection increases the risk of progression to disease in those infected to 7–10% per year.[55a] In addition, individuals previously infected with Mtb may develop disease resulting from exogenous reinfection.[48a,59] This can be readily demonstrated through DNA fingerprinting and is most commonly seen in patients with AIDS.[59]

Medical risk factors for reactivation of tuberculous disease include an abnormal chest radiograph suggestive of previous granulomatous infection, silicosis, diabetes mellitus, prolonged therapy with corticosteroids, other immunosuppressive therapy, reticuloendothelial and hematologic malignancies, end-stage renal disease, oropharyngeal and upper GI malignancies, and being 10% or more below ideal body weight.[6,52]

LABORATORY DIAGNOSIS OF TUBERCULOSIS

The basic diagnostic investigation for tuberculosis includes a medical history, physical examination, skin testing of reactivity to purified protein derivative (PPD), chest x-ray, and collection of relevant biological specimens such as sputum, pleural fluid, urine, stool, blood, cerebrospinal fluid, or biopsy specimens. However, in this section we will focus on the laboratory diagnosis of tuberculosis.

The rapid progression from tuberculosis infection to disease in the context of HIV infection has underscored the need for rapid diagnostic methods. Outbreaks of tuberculosis among persons with AIDS have been associated with a high transmission rate[18] and high case fatality rate[13] in association with delays in initiation of effective therapy.[31] The urgent need for rapid methods for diagnosing tuberculosis is further demonstrated by the enormous difficulty and cost of controlling these outbreaks, particularly when they are due to multidrug-resistant tuberculosis.[34]

While the use of conventional methods such as the acid-fast bacillus (AFB) smear and traditional culture methods remains widespread, newer methods promise to reduce significantly the time to diagnosis of tuberculosis. Additional applications of these evolving technologies include epidemiologic linkage through DNA fingerprinting and rapid determination of drug susceptibility through the luciferase reporter phage system.[41] In this section, we review currently available and emerging technologies for tuberculosis diagnosis and control.

Specimen Collection and Handling

Once pulmonary tuberculosis is suspected, the patient should be instructed to submit a specimen of expectorated sputum. If the patient is unable to expectorate an adequate specimen, sputum induction should be promptly arranged. Once collected, the specimen should be transported immediately to the laboratory. If a long delay is anticipated, the specimen should be refrigerated at 4° C. Nonsterile specimens such as sputum are first subjected to digestion and decontamination, which prevents overgrowth of rapidly growing organisms and concentrates mycobacteria within the specimen. If too vigorous, digestion and decontamination can kill tubercle bacilli. Therefore, quality control programs must ensure that decontamination is sufficiently strong to kill bacteria but not sufficiently strong to kill mycobacteria.[35]

The Acid-fast Smear

Different techniques can be used for the acid-fast test, including the traditional Ziehl-Neelsen stain. The fluorochrome stain uses a fluorescent molecule such as auramine or rhodamine to enable detection of acid-fast organisms. Although it requires more sophistication on the part of the laboratory staff and a fluorescence microscope, the microscopist can screen slides rapidly for acid-fast bacilli. Fluorochrome-positive specimens should be confirmed by traditional techniques.[35] Fluorochrome staining is somewhat more sensitive than the Ziehl-Neelsen stain, but it lacks specificity because the antibody cross-reacts with the cell walls of *Nocardia* and *Corynebacterium*.[35]

The sputum acid-fast stain is accessible, quick, and inexpensive. In the appropriate clinical context it helps narrow the differential diagnosis and it correlates closely with infectiousness. On the other hand, the AFB smear lacks sensitivity. A positive acid-fast smear entails a concentration of at least 10^4 organisms per milliliter. Therefore, this test is more likely to be positive in patients with large bacillary loads: patients with cavitary disease or extensive pulmonary infiltrates.

Another weakness of the AFB stain is its lack of specificity. All mycobacteria, tuberculous and nontuberculous, are acid-fast. In addition, unrelated organisms of the genus *Nocardia* are also weakly acid-fast. Moreover, this test does not discriminate between dead and live organisms and does not by itself establish the presence of active disease.

The use of the acid-fast test should be guided by prior knowledge of the likelihood of disease in the individual tested. For any given diagnostic test, the likelihood of false positive results depends on the sensitivity and specificity of the test and the prevalence of the condition in the population tested. Therefore, to reduce the likelihood of a false positive result, the test should be used when there is reasonable likelihood, even before the test is performed, that disease is present in the person tested.[8] For example, a positive AFB smear is likely to be a true positive in a patient with 3 weeks' cough, a positive tuberculin test, and a right upper lobe cavity. On the other hand, the same result would likely be a false positive in an asymptomatic, HIV seronegative, tuberculin-negative patient with a normal chest x-ray. Therefore, limiting the AFB test to patients with a reasonable chance of having tuberculosis will increase the prevalence of tuberculosis in the population tested and decrease the false positive rate.

Conventional Culture for *Mycobacterium tuberculosis*

Conventional culture is the "gold standard" for the diagnosis of tuberculosis. It is the most commonly used method in the United States. Following digestion and decontamination, sputum specimens are applied directly on an egg-potato base (e.g., Lowenstein-Jensen) and/or agar-base (e.g., Middlebrook 7H-11) solid medium. Growing cultures permit speciation and drug susceptibility testing. Speciation—distinction between *M. tuberculosis* and nontuberculous mycobacteria such as *Mycobacterium avium-intracellulare*—is based on the rate of growth, physical characteristics, and results of a series of standard biochemical assays. This method is most sensitive and reliable when tubercle bacilli are in concentrations of at least 10^3 organisms per milliliter, and it can be used for any type of specimen, including blood, urine, cerebrospinal fluid, pleural fluid, or peritoneal fluid.

Using this culture method, it usually takes approximately 4–12 weeks for cultures to be identified positive and several more weeks for sensitivity testing. In addition, this test requires a reasonably well-equipped laboratory. The delays associated with conventional culture methods have encouraged the development of newer methods for rapid diagnosis of tuberculosis.

The BACTEC TB System

Radiometric methods such as the BACTEC system depend on the growth of mycobacteria in ^{14}C-labeled palmitic acid as substrate in liquid medium. As the organisms metabolize this substrate, they release $^{14}CO_2$, which provides a quantitative measure of mycobacterial growth.[43,57]

The BACTEC system for tuberculosis diagnosis has several advantages. It is widely available and can indicate mycobacterial growth weeks before conventional cultures on solid medium. In a multicenter study, organism growth could be detected within 8 days by the BACTEC system versus 18 days by conventional media.[55] Similarly, organism growth from smear-negative specimens could be detected within an average of 14 days with the BACTEC media vesus 26 days with conventional media.[45] In addition, *M. tuberculosis* complex can be easily identified by the NAP test, an assay that consists of the addition of an intermediate of chloramphenicol (NAP, or *p*-nitro-alpha-acetylamino-beta-hydroxyropiophenone) that inhibits the growth of *M. tuberculosis* but not other mycobacteria. Thus, speciation of mycobacteria can be accomplished in a few days.

Using the BACTEC system, it is possible to identify growing mycobacteria in 1 week and to identify mycobacteria as *M. tuberculosis* or other species by the NAP test within 5 additional days.[35] As in conventional culture, the speed of identification of mycobacteria depends on the concentration in the initial inoculum.[56] When combined with a DNA probe for an Mtb-specific rRNA sequence, radiometric culture methods allow for identification of *M. tuberculosis* in 1–3 weeks.[16,28] In addition, this system provides for easier recovery of mycobacteria in AFB-negative sputum specimens and other body fluids, including blood, urine, and stool. Moreover, this system is easily adapted for drug susceptibility testing, thereby resulting in additional time savings.[57]

Assays of Mycolic Acid Pattern

Large amounts of lipids are present in the mycobacterial cell wall, and the potential use of these lipids in the diagnosis of tuberculosis is under investigation. Methods used to separate mycolic acid residues using chromatographic methods include high-performance liquid chromatography, thin-layer chromatography, and gas-liquid chromatography. The mycolic acid pattern obtained with chromatography is species-specific and reproducible.[35]

The test for tuberculostearic acid (TSA) is the most commonly used chromatographic technique.[32,49] This fatty acid is produced by almost all species belonging to the genera *Mycobacteria* and *Nocardia.* In addition, oropharyngeal commensal flora contain *Actinomyces* organisms, whose cell wall includes TSA. However, despite its apparent lack of specificity, when this test is positive in cerebrospinal fluid, it is highly indicative of tuberculous meningitis, particularly in areas where the prevalence of nontuberculous mycobacteria is low. Indeed, detection of TSA in serum and cerebrospinal fluid has been suggested as a means to rapidly diagnose tuberculous meningitis. Detection of TSA by high-performance liquid chromatography requires only 8 hours; it is more sensitive than the acid-fast smear and nearly as sensitive as conventional culture.[33a]

However, this technique is limited by the requirement for 10^7–10^8 tubercle bacilli: growing cultures for several weeks. In addition, this assay requires the use of expensive equipment that is available only in highly specialized laboratories.[11]

Immunodiagnosis of *Mycobacterium tuberculosis*

Currently, immunodiagnostic methods such as enzyme-linked immunosorbent assays (ELISA), immunoelectrophoresis, hemagglutination assays, fluorescent antibodies, and radioimmunoassays are not used routinely in the clinical diagnosis of tuberculosis. However, ELISA methods have the potential to enhance the diagnostic work-up for tuberculosis in certain situations, particularly tuberculous meningitis.

ENZYME-LINKED IMMUNOSORBENT ASSAYS

Detection of* M. tuberculosis *antigens. Detection of mycobacterial antigens by ELISA in sputum is problematic because most soluble antigens are discarded or denatured during digestion and decontamination of sputum specimens. Nonetheless, in two small series,[2,42] the sensitivity of antigen detection was 76%–89%. The specificity of these tests could not be ascertained because sputa of patients with nontuberculous mycobacterial disease were not studied. ELISA or RIA methods are superior to acid-fast stains in the diagnosis of tuberculous meningitis, where the cerebrospinal fluid (CSF) typically harbors a low concentration of mycobacteria.[51,66] In the ELISA, antibodies to mycobacterial antigens are first added to microtiter wells and become plastic-bound. When CSF mycobacterial antigens from the specimen become bound specifically to the active site of the plastic-bound antibody, the antigen-antibody complex can then be detected by addition of a second antimycobacterial antibody that is linked to an enzyme that produces a color change after addition of appropriate substrate. Radioimmunoassay for mycobacterial antigens in CSF has variable sensitivity, 39%–79%, and high specificity, 98%–100%.[51,66]

Detection of Antimycobacterial Antibodies. ELISA also can be used to detect antimycobacterial antibodies in serum and other body fluids. For this assay, microtiter wells are coated with mycobacterial antigen, and patient sera are added to these wells containing plastic-bound antigens. This results in binding human antimycobacterial antibodies to these antigens. This is followed by linking human immunoglobulin antibodies to an enzyme that catalyzes a color reaction upon addition of appropriate substrate.

In one study, the sputum acid-fast stain achieved greater sensitivity and specificity than serodiagnosis by ELISA. Stain was 79% sensitive and 100% specific; ELISA, 69% sensitive and 88% specific.[20] Moreover, in smear-negative tuberculosis, a lower bacillary burden is thought to trigger less antibody production, thus reducing the sensitivity of antibody detection in serum.[15] Similarly, in people with AIDS the sensitivity of serodiagnosis is reduced, presumably because of diminished antibody production.[63]

Use of ELISA in serodiagnosis of tuberculosis, like the sputum acid-fast stain, is most likely to be sensitive in patients with large bacillary burdens. In this setting, the combination of ELISA with results of first flourochrome sputum resulted in a sensitivity of 86%. When both tests were negative, the negative predictive value was 97%.[67]

On the other hand, in populations with a low prevalence of tuberculosis, as with the acid-fast smear, the utility of the ELISA technique in the diagnosis of tuberculosis is reduced by a substantial rate of false positive results. Differences in the antigen used and the types of control populations studied also contribute to this lack of specificity.

RAPID *M. TUBERCULOSIS* IDENTIFICATION TESTS

Techniques for rapid identification of *M. tuberculosis* usually require substantial mycobacterial growth before speciation is possible. Within this category are the NAP test, assays based on detection of mycolic acid patterns, assays of genetic homology with mycobacterium tuberculosis, and DNA fingerprinting. However, amplification of mycobacterial DNA through the polymerase chain reaction, combined with speciation using specific probes, brings the goal of rapid diagnosis and epidemiologic linkage clearly within our reach.

DNA-based Techniques and Applications

Determination of Genetic Homology

Once mycobacterial cultures have grown, nucleic acids can be extracted and purified and speciation performed based on homology to known sequences of mycobacterial ribosomal RNA. The mycobacterial genome consists of only one chromosome. However, each *M. tuberculosis* cell carries approximately 10,000 ribosomes. Therefore, targeting ribosomal RNA increases the sensitivity of assays of homology 10^4 times. Specifically, single-stranded DNA oligonucleotide probes labeled with chemiluminescent acridium are directed against these ribosomal RNA sequences, and the labeled hybrid molecules are detected by a luminometer. Speciation of *M. tuberculosis* is made possible by the high specificity of this hybridization. However, because of the extensive (94–97%) homology between the nucleic acids of *M. tuberculosis* and those of *Mycobacterium africanum* and *Mycobacterium bovis*, this assay does not differentiate between these species. Therefore, the result of this test is reported as *Mtb complex* and not distinguished from *M. bovis* or *M. africanum*. Nevertheless, since the latter two species seldom occur in the United States, a report of *Mtb complex* reliably reflects the detection of *M. tuberculosis*.

POLYMERASE CHAIN REACTION

One major limitation of all techniques described thus far for identification of *M. tuberculosis* is the requirement for growth of sufficient organisms. The polymerase chain reaction (PCR) promises to substantially reduce the time to diagnosis of tuberculosis in clinical specimens through rapid amplification of mycobacterial DNA followed by speciation using specific DNA probes.

Through PCR, it is possible to amplify mycobacterial DNA 10^6 times in 1–2 days. Several DNA sequences that are specific to Mtb are known, including the putative insertion sequence IS6110,[26,27,36] those that encode ribosomal RNA,[7] and the sequences that encode some key mycobacterial antigens.[9,23,50] Most PCR-based assays consist of amplification of specific *known* sequences of mycobacterial DNA in clinical samples followed by separation of DNA segments by gel electrophoresis. Commonly used PCR-based assays involve transfer of the PCR product to nylon membranes, followed by hybridization to oligonucleotide probes that specifically bind DNA from *M. tuberculosis*. When radiolabeled probes are used, incorporation of radioactivity indicates a positive result. With enzyme-linked probes, hybridization to mycobacterial DNA is detected through colorimetric assays. A new PCR-based method separates the PCR products by polyacrylamide gel electrophoresis. The gel is then stained with ethidium bromide, and a positive result is easily recognized as a band of expected molecular weight.[26,27] Using this assay, Eisenach et al. reported 100% sensitivity in 46 smear-positive sputum samples from patients with tuberculosis and 99% specificity in 68 samples from non-tuberculous patients.[27]

Despite their potential to reduce the time to diagnosis of tuberculosis substantially, PCR-based methods pose significant technical challenges. During DNA amplification, cross-contamination with airborne PCR products may lead to false positive results. Contamination of reagents with DNA from *M. tuberculosis* is another potential problem, and great caution must be exercised to confirm recovery of sufficient amounts of mycobacterial DNA in each reaction mixture.[27]

DNA FINGERPRINTING AND MOLECULAR EPIDEMIOLOGY

To prove transmission of Mtb from one person to another, one must provide evidence that a susceptible host was exposed to a specific strain of *M. tuberculosis* from an individual with active tuberculosis and subsequently became infected with the same strain of *M. tuberculosis*. Though organisms of the same strain usually have the same drug susceptibility, drug sensitivity is not strain-specific. Moreover, same-strain organisms may have different drug sensitivity profiles, which typically occurs in patients who develop secondary drug resistance because they did not adhere to therapy; that is, the same strain acquires a new drug susceptibility profile.

The genome of Mtb consists of a single circular chromosome containing 2.1 Kb of DNA. Like other bacteria, the genome of Mtb contains insertion sequences, also known as transposable elements. These highly conserved sequences of DNA vary in number and location in different strains of bacteria.[12,36,37] Insertion sequence 6110 (IS6110) is well characterized, and molecular epidemiologic studies of tuberculosis are based on its location and number within specific strains. Most strains of *M. tuberculosis* contain 6–15 copies of insertion sequence 6110 (IS 6110) (range 2–20).[16,65] The nucleotide sequence of IS6110 includes one single site each for the restriction enzymes Pvu II and BamH1. By convention, only the Pvu II site is used for strain typing.

DNA fingerprinting involves extraction and purification of mycobacterial DNA, followed by digestion with Pvu II. Since the mycobacterial genome is circular, the number of segments of DNA following Pvu II digest is equal to the number of Pvu II sites within the specific strain of Mtb. Similarly, the length of each segment thus obtained depends on the distance between insertion sequences in that particular strain. Consequently, differences (polymorphism) are expected in the lengths of fragments of DNA that are generated by digestion of different strains of *M. tuberculosis* with the restriction enzyme Pvu II—hence the term *restriction fragment length polymorphism* (RFLP). The resulting segments of DNA can then be separated on the basis of molecular size by agarose gel electrophoresis and then transferred onto nitrocellulose. Probing this nitrocellulose membrane with radiolabeled oligonucleotide sequences that are complementary to the nucleotide sequence on either side of this Pvu II site will result in hybridization with the specific DNA sequences that are known to flank the Pvu II site of IS6110. Since the length of the segments varies according to the number and location of these insertion sequences in a given strain, a highly specific pattern can be detected upon probing a specific strain. Hence the term *DNA fingerprinting* is now in usage.

Since probing for both sides that flank the Pvu II site would yield too many bands on the gel and thus reduce resolution, standardized methods for DNA fingerprinting only probe one side of the DNA segments resulting from Pvu II digest.[64] Computerized databases of DNA fingerprints are being developed based on standards adopted between laboratories in North America and Europe. These databases will allow comparison of DNA fingerprints for Mtb within and between populations.[64] RFLP analysis (or DNA fingerprinting, or strain typing) has emerged as an important tool in studies of the molecular epidemiology of *M. tuberculosis.*

In investigations of outbreaks, distinct DNA fingerprints are observed in strains of Mtb from tuberculosis patients who are not epidemiologically linked. On the other hand, given a common source of Mtb, identical DNA fingerprints were detected in all isolates from tuberculosis patients of the same household or congregate facility.[18,24,25] The DNA fingerprint is stable following development of drug resistance[59,65] and after culture for 2–6 months.[37,65] Occasionally, an additional DNA fragment is observed in some isolates from a given outbreak, or after culture for a prolonged time.[59] While this presumably indicates replication of IS6110 during disease transmission, it usually does not cause a practical problem in epidemiologic linkage of tuberculosis because the overall DNA banding pattern is similar. Thus, DNA fingerprints of individual Mtb strains remain relatively stable over time and permit definitive delineation of patterns of tuberculosis transmission.

This technique has already yielded valuable insights into the rapid progression of tuberculosis in patients with AIDS. In addition, it has provided solid evidence for exogenous reinfection as an important pathogenetic mechanism in patients whose treatment was failing despite appropriate therapy for tuberculosis.[59] However, because DNA fingerprinting requires significant amounts of DNA, it is limited to culture-positive cases. Another limitation is that RFLP analysis cannot be used to track specific strains in PPD-positive converters.

New strategies that remain to be translated into clinical practice will combine PCR with DNA fingerprinting for rapid identification of *M. tuberculosis* based on detection of IS6110. With this combination, it is anticipated that the RFLP pattern will sometimes be the first clue that a patient may have a multidrug-resistant strain of *M. tuberculosis*—several weeks before conventional culture results. This information will be extremely valuable in efforts to prevent nosocomial transmission of tuberculosis.

While DNA fingerprinting is a powerful technology, its routine application to epidemiologic studies of tuberculosis is currently undergoing a rigorous evaluation. Until the promises and pitfalls of this technology are better characterized, it remains a tool without routine clinical application. Moreover, conclusions about spread of tuberculosis based on DNA fingerprinting must be consistent with data obtained through contact investigation—so-called "shoe-leather epidemiology."

CONCLUSION

Tuberculosis is preventable, and its pathogenesis is generally well understood. The resurgence of this disease in epidemic proportions has significantly increased the risk of occupational exposure among workers who are likely to come into contact with individuals with infectious tuberculosis. On the other hand, it is now possible that emerging molecular techniques, including DNA-based technologies, will help reduce the risk of occupational exposure if they are applied judiciously. Such reduction would be possible through a reduction in exposure time, more rapid and definitive identification of outbreaks, and more rapid control. The challenge today is to critically evaluate these emerging technologies and determine their application in public health practice.

REFERENCES

1. Alland D, Kalkut GE, Moss AR, et al: Transmission of tuberculosis in New York City: An analysis by DNA fingerprinting and conventional epidemiologic methods. N Engl J Med 330:1710–1716, 1994.
2. Al-Orainey IO, El Rab MOG, Al-Hajjaj MS, Saeed ES: Detection of mycobacterial antigens in sputum by an enzyme immunoassay. Eur J Clin Microbiol Infect Dis 11:58–61, 1992.
3. Barsdale L, Kim KS: Mycobacterium. Bacteriol Rev 41:217–372, 1977.
4. Bates JH: Tuberculosis: Susceptibilty and resistance. Am Rev Respir Dis 125:20–24, 1982.
5. Beck-Sague C, Dooley SW, Hutton MD, et al: Hospital outbreak of multi-drug-resistant Mycobacterium tuberculosis infection: Factors in transmission to staff and HIV-infected patients. JAMA 268:1280–1286, 1992.
6. Bloch AB, Rieder HL, Kelly GD, et al: The epidemiology of tuberculosis in the United States. Implications for diagnosis and treatment. Clin Chest Med 10:297–313, 1989.
7. Boddinghaus B, Rogall T, Flohr T, et al: Detection and identification of mycobacteria by amplification of rRNA. J Clin Microbiol 28:1751–1759, 1990.
8. Boyd JC, Marr JJ: Decreasing reliability of acid-fast smear techniques for detection of tuberculosis. Ann Intern Med 92:489–492, 1975.
9. Brisson-Noel A, Aznar C, Chureau C, et al: Diagnosis of tuberculosis by DNA amplification in clinical practice evaluation. Lancet 338:364–366, 1991.
10. Brudney K, Dobkin J: Resurgent tuberculosis in New York City. Am Rev Respir Dis 144:745–749, 1991.
11. Butler WR, Kilburn JO: Identification of major slowly growing pathogenic mycobacteria and Mycobacterium gordonae by high performance liquid chromatography of their mycolic acids. J Clin Microbiol 26:50–53, 1988.
12. Cave MD, Eisenach KD, McDermott PF, et al: IS 6110: Conservation of sequence in Mycobacterium tuberculosis complex and its utilization in DNA fingerprinting. Mol Cell Probes 5:73–80, 1991.
13. Centers for Disease Control: Nosocomial transmission of multidrug-resistant tuberculosis among HIV-infected persons—Florida and New York, 1988–91. MMWR 40:585–591, 1991.

14. Centers for Disease Control: Tuberculosis morbidity in the United States: 1990. Final data. MMWR 40(SS-3):23–28, 1992.
15. Chan SL, Reggiardo Z, Daniel TM, et al: Serodiagnosis of tuberculosis using an ELISA with antigen 5 and hemagglutination assay with glycolipid antigens. Am Rev Respir Dis 142:385–390, 1990.
16. Crawford JT, Eisenach KD, Bates JH: Diagnosis of tuberculosis: Present and future. Semin Respir Infect 4:171–181, 1989.
17. Crowle AJ, Elkins N: Relative permissiveness of macrophages from black and white people for virulent tubercle bacilli. Infect Immun 58:632–638, 1990.
18. Daley CL, Small PM, Schecter GF, et al: An outbreak of tuberculosis with accelerated progression among persons infected with human immunodeficiency virus: An analysis using restriction fraction length polymorphysims. N Engl J Med 326:231–325, 1992.
19. Daniel TM, DeBanne SM: The serodiagnosis of tuberculosis and other mycobacterial diseases by enzyme-linked immunosorbent assay. Am Rev Respir Dis 135:1137–1151, 1987.
20. Daniel TM, De Murillo GL, Sawyer JA, et al: Field evaluation of enzyme-linked immunosorbent assay for the serodiagnosis of tuberculosis. Am Rev Respir Dis 134:662–665, 1986.
21. Dannenberg AM: Delayed-type hypersensitivity and cell-mediated immunity in the pathogenesis of tuberculosis. Immunol Today 12:228–233, 1991.
22. Dannenberg AM: Pathogenesis of pulmonary tuberculosis: Host-parasite interactions cell-mediated immunity, and delayed-type hypersensitivity. In Schlossberg D (ed): Basic Principles in Tuberculosis. 3rd ed. New York, Springer-Verlag, 1992.
23. Del Portillo P, Murillo LA, Patarroyo ME: Amplification of a species-specific DNA fragment of Mycobacterium tuberculosis and its possible use in diagnosis. J Clin Microbiol 29:2163–2168, 1991.
24. Dooley SW, Villarino ME, Lawrence M, et al: Nosocomial transmission of tuberculosis in a hospital unit for HIV-infected patients. JAMA 267:2632–2635, 1991.
25. Edlin BR, Tokars JI, Gieco MH, et al: An outbreak of multidrug-resistant tuberculosis among hospitalized patients with the acquired immunodeficiency syndrome. N Engl J Med 326:1514–1521, 1992.
26. Eisenach KD, Cave D, Bates JH, Crawford JT: Polymerase chain reaction amplification of a repetitive DNA sequence specific for Mycobacterium tuberculosis. J Infect Dis 161:977–981, 1990.
27. Eisenach KD, Sifford MD, Cave MD, et al: Detection of Mycobacterium tuberculosis in sputum samples using a polymerase chain reaction. Am Rev Respir Dis 144:1660–1163, 1991.
28. Ellner PD, Kighn TE, Commerata R, Hosmer M: Rapid detection and identification of pathogenic mycobacteria by combining radiometric and nucleic acid probe methods. J Clin Microbiol 26:1349–1352, 1988.
29. Felton CP, Ford JG: Tuberculosis in the inner city. In Reichman LB, Hershfield ES (eds): Tuberculosis: A Comprehensive International Approach. Lung Biology in Health and Disease series, Vol 66. New York, Marcel Dekker, 1993, pp 483–503.
30. Felton CP, Smith JA, Ehrlich MH: Racial differences and Mycobacterium tuberculosis infection [letter]. N Engl J Med 322:1670–1671, 1990.
31. Fischl MA, Uttamchandani RB, Daikos GL, et al: An outbreak of tuberculosis caused by multiple-drug-resistant tubercle bacilli in patients with HIV infection. Ann Intern Med 117:177–183, 1992.
32. French GL, Chan CY, Cheung SW, Oo KT: Diagnosis of pulmonary tuberculosis by detection of tuberculostearic acid in sputum by using gas chromatography-mass spectrometry with selected ion monitoring. J Infect Dis 156:356–362, 1987.
33. Frieden TR, Sterling T, Pablos-Mendez A, et al: The emergence of multidrug-resistant tuberculosis in New York City. N Engl J Med 328:521–526, 1993.
33a. Glassroth J: Diagnosis of tuberculosis. In Reichman LB, Hershfield ES (eds): Tuberculosis: A Comprehensive International Approach. Lung Biology in Health and Disease series, Vol 66. New York, Marcel Dekker, 1993, pp 149–166.
34. Goble M, Iseman MD, Madsen LA, et al: Treatment of 171 patients with pulmonary tuberculosis resistant to isoniazid and rifampin. N Engl J Med 328:527–532, 1993.
35. Grosset JH: Bacteriology of tuberculosis. In Reichman LB, Hershfield ES (eds): Tuberculosis: A Comprehensive International Approach. Lung Biology in Health and Disease series, Vol 66. New York, Marcel Dekker, 1993, pp 49–74.
36. Hermans PWM, Schuitema ARJ, van Soolingen D, et al: Specific detection of Mycobacterium tuberculosis complex strains by polymerase chain reaction. J Clin Microbiol 28:1204–1213, 1990.

37. Hermans PWM, Van Soolingen D, Dale JW, et al: Insertion element IS 986 from Mycobacterium tuberculosis: A useful tool for diagnosis and epidemiology of tuberculosis. J Clin Microbiol 28:2051–2058, 1990.
38. Hoge CW, Fisher L, Donnell HD Jr, et al: Risk factors for transmission of Mycobacterium tuberculosis in a primary school: Lack of racial difference in susceptibility to infection. Am J Epidemiol 139:520–530, 1994.
39. Hoge CW, Fisher L, Donnell HD Jr, et al: Reply to "Invited commentary: Relative susceptibility of black Americans to tuberculosis" [editorial]. Am J Epidemiol 139:533–534, 1994.
40. Hopewell PC: Tuberculosis and infection with HIV. In Reichman LB, Hershfield ES (eds): Tuberculosis: A Comprehensive International Approach. Lung Biology in Health and Disease series, Vol 66. New York, Marcel Dekker, 1993, pp 369–394.
41. Jacobs WR Jr, Barletta RG, Udani R, et al: Rapid assessment of drug susceptibilities of Mycobacterium tuberculosis by means of Luciferase reporter phages. Science 260:819–822, 1993.
42. Kansal R, Khuller GK: Detection of mannophosphoinositide antigens in sputum of tuberculosis patients by dot enzyme immunoassay. Med Microbiol Immunol 180:73–78, 1991.
43. Middlebrook G, Reggiardo Z, Tigerdt WD: Automable radiometric detection of growth of Mycobacterium tuberculosis in selective media. Am Rev Respir Dis 115:1066–1069, 1977.
44. Minnikin DE: Lipids: Complex lipids, their chemistry, biosynthesis and roles. In Rutledge C, Stanford J (eds): The Biology of Mycobacteria, Vol 1, Sec 3. London, Academic Press, 1982, pp 95–184.
45. Morgan MS, Horstmeier CD, De Young DR, Roberts GD: Comparison of a radiometric method (BACTEC) and conventional culture media for recovery of mycobacteria from smear-negative specimens. J Clin Microbiol 18:384–388, 1983.
46. Murray JF, Nadel JA: Textbook of Respiratory Medicine. Philadelphia, WB Saunders, 1988.
47. Nardell EA: Pathogenesis of tuberculosis. In Reichman LB, Hershfield ES (eds): Tuberculosis: A Comprehensive International Approach. Lung Biology in Health and Disease series, Vol 66. New York, Marcel Dekker, 1993, pp 103–122..
48. Nardell EA, Keegan J, Cheney SA, Etkind SC: Airborne infection: Theoretical limits of protection achievable by building ventilation. Am Rev Respir Dis 144:302–306, 1991.
48a. Nardell E, McInnis B, Thomas S: Exogenous reinfection with tuberculosis in a shelter for the homeless. N Engl J Med 315:1570–1575, 1986.
49. Pang JA, Chan HS, Chan CY, et al: A tuberculostearic acid assay in the diagnosis of sputum smear-negative tuberculosis. A prospective study of bronchoscopic aspirate and lavage specimens. Ann Intern Med 111:650–654, 1989.
50. Pao CC, Yen TSB, You JB, et al: Detection and identification of Mycobacterium tuberculosis by DNA amplification. J Clin Microbiol 28:1877–1880, 1990.
51. Radhakrishman VV, Mathai A: Detection of Mycobacterium tuberculosis antigen 5 in cerebrospinal fluid by inhibition ELISA and its diagnostic potential in tuberculous meningitis. J Infect Dis 163:650–652, 1991.
52. Rieder HL, Cauthen GM, Comstock GW, Snider DE Jr: Epidemiology of tuberculosis in the United States. Epidemiol Rev 11:79–98, 1989.
53. Riley RL: Transmission and environmental control of tuberculosis. In Reichman LB, Hershfield ES (eds): Tuberculosis: A Comprehensive International Approach. Lung Biology in Health and Disease series, Vol 66. New York, Marcel Dekker, 1993, pp 123–136.
54. Riley RL, Mills CC, O'Grady F: Infectiousness of air from a tuberculosis ward. Am Rev Respir Dis 85:511–525, 1962.
55. Roberts GD, Koneman EW, Kim YK: Mycobacterium. In Hausler WJ Jr, Herrman KL, Isenberg HD, Shadomy HJ (eds): Manual of Clinical Microbiology. 5th ed. Washington, DC, American Society for Microbiology, 1991, pp 304–309.
55a. Selwyn PA, Hartel D, Lewis VA, et al: A prospective study of the risk of tuberculosis among intravenous drug users with human immunodeficiency virus infection. N Engl J Med 320:545–550, 1989.
56. Siddiqui SH, Hwangbo CC, Silcox V, et al: Rapid radiometric methods to detect and differentiate Mycobacterium tuberculosis/bovis from other mycobacterial species. Am Rev Respir Dis 130:634–640, 1984.
57. Siddiqui SH, Libonati JP, Middlebrook G: Evaluation of a rapid radiometric method for drug susceptibility testing of Mycobacterium tuberculosis. J Clin Microbiol 13:908–912, 1981.
58. Small PM, Hopewell PC, Singh SP, et al: The epidemiology of tuberculosis in San Francisco: A population based study using conventional and molecular methods. N Engl J Med 330:1703–1709, 1994.

59. Small PM, Shafer RW, Hopewell PC, et al: Exogenous reinfection with multidrug-resistant tuberculosis in patients with advanced HIV infection. N Engl J Med 328:1137–1144, 1993.
60. Smith DW: Diseases in guinea pigs. In Kubica GP, Wayne LG (eds): The Mycobacteria, Part G. New York, Marcel Dekker, 1984, pp 925–946.
61. Stead WW, Lofgren JP, Senner JW: Invited commentary: Relative susceptibility of black Americans to tuberculosis. Am J Epidemiol 139:531–532, 1994.
62. Stead WW, Senner JW, Reddick WT, Lofgren JP: Racial differences in susceptibility to infection by Mycobacterium tuberculosis. N Engl J Med 322:422–427, 1990.
63. Van der Werf TS, Das PK, Van Soolingen D, et al: Sero-diagnosis of tuberculosis with A60 antigen enzyme-linked immunosorbent assay: Failure in HIV-infected individuals in Ghana. Med Microbiol Immunol 181:71–76, 1992.
64. Van Embden JDA, Cave MD, Crawford JT, et al: Strain identification of Mycobacterium tuberculosis by DNA fingerprinting: Recommendation for a standardized methodology. J Clin Microbiol 31:406–409, 1993.
65. Van Soolingen D, Hermans PWM, de Haas PEW, et al: Occurrence and stability of insertion sequences in Mycobacterium tuberculosis complex strains: Evaluation of an insertion sequence-dependent DNA polymorphism as a tool in the epidemiology of tuberculosis. J Clin Microbiol 29:2578–2586, 1991.
66. Watt G, Zaraspe G, Bautista S, Laughlin LW: Rapid diagnosis of tuberculous meningitis by using an enzyme-linked immunosorbent assay to detect mycobacterial antigen and antibody in cerebrospinal fluid. J Infect Dis 158:681–686, 1988.
67. Zeiss CR, Kalish SB, Erlich KS, et al: IgG antibody to purified protein derivative by enzyme-linked immunosorbent assay in the diagnosis of pulmonary tuberculosis. Am Rev Respir Dis 130:845–848, 1984.

DAVID N. ROSE, MD

THE RELATIONSHIP BETWEEN TB AND HIV INFECTIONS

From the AIDS Center
Mount Sinai Hospital
New York, New York

Reprint requests to:
David N. Rose, MD
Box 1009
Mount Sinai Medical Center
New York, NY 10029

The increase in reported cases of tuberculosis since the mid 1980s is variously attributed to the growth in poverty, homelessness and drug abuse, the defunding of TB control programs, increased immigration from high-prevalence countries, and the acquired immunodeficiency syndrome (AIDS) epidemic.[1,5,8,45] Although the relative contributions and the interrelationships of these are not known, AIDS is widely believed to be the strongest influence. Recent evidence suggests that AIDS has substantially undermined the nation's strategic plan to eliminate TB in the United States.[12,13,62] Globally and nationally, the growth of TB parallels the growth of AIDS. The diminished cell-mediated immunity caused by the human immunodeficiency virus (HIV) is now considered to be the most powerful risk factor for the activation of latent *Mycobacterium tuberculosis* infection.[62] Furthermore, people infected with HIV have been found to be especially susceptible to newly acquired *M. tuberculosis* disease. TB outbreaks have been recently reported in institutional settings such as hospitals and correctional facilities, with alarmingly high case-fatality rates.[7,22,35,41,65,83] HIV infection played a prominent role in these outbreaks.

In several important ways, TB risks in the workplace are made worse by the AIDS epidemic. In addition to the high TB risks among HIV-infected people, TB also threatens people who are not infected with HIV. It is one of the few contagious diseases of AIDS that patients spread in the workplace. Airborne droplet transmission of tubercle bacilli to workers is made more likely by the special features of TB in

HIV-infected people. This chapter reviews the unique interrelationship and the epidemiology, pathogenesis, clinical manifestations, prevention, and treatment of these two infections.

THE OVERLAPPING AIDS AND TB EPIDEMICS

One third of the world's population, 1.7 billion people, are infected with *M. tuberculosis*. In 1990, an estimated 8 million new cases of TB occurred worldwide, 95% in developing nations and 5% in industrialized countries. Most of this disease, 63%, occurred in Southeast Asia and the western Pacific. Africa accounted for an additional 17% of the world's TB cases; 7% occurred in the Americas, 8% in eastern Mediterranean countries, and 5% in Europe.[50] TB caused approximately 2.9 million deaths worldwide in 1990,[50] and among infectious diseases it is the leading cause of death.[5] It is estimated that 30–60% of adults in developing countries[47] and 10–15 million people in the United States are infected with *M. tuberculosis*.[15]

In 1991, 10 million people worldwide had HIV infection, by World Health Organization estimates.[55] In contrast to TB, Africa carries the largest burden of HIV, with approximately 6 million infected people. An estimated 2 million people are infected in the Americas, 1 million in Asia and Oceania, and 0.5 million in Europe.[55] An estimated 1.5 million people worldwide have died from AIDS.[5] Approximately 1 million people in the United States are infected with HIV. As of March 1993, 289,320 AIDS cases had been reported to the Centers for Disease Control and Prevention (CDC).[26]

The extent of overlap between people infected with *M. tuberculosis* and HIV is not fully known and probably varies from locality to locality. The manifestation of the overlapping epidemics, nevertheless, is made obvious by the changing TB epidemic. The three-decade decline in TB in the United States ceased in 1984, with 22,255 reported cases that year. In 1992, 26,673 cases were reported,[25] a 20% increase since 1984. The growth follows and parallels the growth of the AIDS epidemic.

Several epidemiologic phenomena suggest that AIDS is an important cause of the resurgence of TB.[1] First, TB has increased most in cities and states with the highest AIDS rates. States with the highest incidence of AIDS in 1990 (District of Columbia, New York, New Jersey, Florida, and California) also had the highest rate of deaths with TB, 2.82 per 100,000 people age 20–49. In these states and in this age group, the rate rose 362% between 1982 and 1990. In contrast, in the same age group the rate of deaths with TB rose 47% in states with a low incidence of AIDS and 52% in states with a medium incidence of AIDS.[6] This is most conspicuous in New York City, the city with the greatest number of reported AIDS cases.[26] Among New Yorkers of all ages, TB cases increased 132% in the 1980s and 32% between 1989 and 1990.[88]

Second, the demographic groups at the highest risk of AIDS also have the highest increases in the incidence of TB.[23] In past decades, most TB cases occurred among the elderly.[75] In recent years, a noticeable increase in reported cases occurred among people age 25–44,[75] the peak age of the AIDS epidemic.[23] Between 1985 and 1990, the largest increases in TB cases occurred among men age 25–44,[23] a group that also accounted for 68.4% of all AIDS cases reported to the CDC as of 1990.[26] A recent study of death certificates by the National Center for Health Statistics confirms this. The age distribution of TB deaths in the United States changed between 1980, when the peak of deaths occurred in people age 70–74, and 1990, when the peak of deaths in the elderly was accompanied by a second peak in people age 20–44.[7] Furthermore, in the 1980s, TB increased among Hispanics by 54.7% and among non-Hispanic blacks by 26.9%, but decreased by 7.3% among non-Hispanic whites.[20]

Third, between 1984 and 1989, extrapulmonary TB increased by 20% while pulmonary TB increased by 3%.[1] High rates of extrapulmonary TB are characteristic of TB in AIDS patients.[1,9,10] Fourth, HIV-infected people are more likely to develop primary disease shortly after *M. tuberculosis* infection than people not infected with HIV.[33,35] Furthermore, HIV-infected people with long-standing latent *M. tuberculosis* infection, as evidenced by a positive tuberculin skin test, are far more likely than uninfected people to develop active TB each year.[61,78] Most cases of TB among HIV-infected people are believed to result from reactivation of latent *M. tuberculosis* infection rather than newly acquired infection.

Finally, TB is especially common among AIDS patients. Early reports in the AIDS epidemic found active TB among AIDS patients in Haiti[70] and among Haitian and non-Haitian patients in south Florida.[73] In Africa, TB is considered to be the most common HIV-associated lung disease[45] and one of the most common opportunistic infections.[47] In a hospital in Madrid, more than 60% of AIDS patients had TB during the course of their illness.[61] In a registry matching study in the United States, 4% of AIDS cases were found to also appear on TB registries; 5% of AIDS patients in New York City and 10% in Florida also had TB.[13] Marked racial differences were found in Florida: 2% of non-Hispanic whites, 7% of Hispanics, 15% of U.S.-born blacks, and 29% of Haitians with AIDS also had TB.[75] The association between TB and AIDS is also particularly high among intravenous drug users.[13] TB is increasingly associated with death among AIDS patients. In 1987, 2.3% of AIDS patients who died in the United States also had TB. In 1990, 3.0% had TB.[6] These rates were especially pronounced among blacks and Hispanics. Between 1987 and 1990, the proportion of deaths in people with AIDS and TB rose from 3.8% to 4.7% among blacks and Hispanics, but only from 1.3% to 1.6% among whites.[6]

Similarly, HIV infection is commonly found among TB patients. A total of 38% of the TB patients in a sanitarium and 17% of the patients in an outpatient TB diagnostic center in Kinshasa, Zaire, where seropositive for HIV.[30] Two thirds of the TB patients in a Kampala, Uganda, hospital[39] and 60% of the TB patients in a Lusaka, Zambia, hospital were found to be HIV-seropositive.[38] In the United States, HIV infection was found in 31% of TB patients in Miami,[73] 23% in Seattle,[66] and 28% in San Francisco.[87] In a 1988–1989 seroprevalence study conducted by the Centers for Disease Control (CDC) in 20 TB clinics nationwide, HIV infection was found in 0–46.3% (median 3.4%) of the clinics' 3,077 TB patients. HIV prevalence rates were highest in the Northeast and Atlantic coastal areas, in people born in the United States, Haiti or Cuba, and in people age 30–39.[68] Among TB patients in Miami, HIV prevalence rates were highest among blacks and Haitians and in the age group 25–44.[73]

PATHOGENESIS OF *MYCOBACTERIUM TUBERCULOSIS* AND HIV CO-INFECTIONS

Cellular immunity is the sole host defense against TB. Although a variety of antibodies are produced following *M. tuberculosis* infection, humoral immunity is not known to play a role in TB control. Host defense mechanisms in the first weeks following ingestion or inhalation of the tubercle bacillus require intact macrophage and T-lymphocyte function. Cutaneous delayed-type hypersensitivity (DTH), granuloma formation, and tissue necrosis develop within 6–14 weeks. If the tubercle bacilli are not destroyed, they multiply and are retained in macrophages. What follows depends upon an interplay of immunologic mediators still not fully understood: either primary TB disease or a latent infection of variable duration and the risk of "adult" TB disease.

HIV infects and/or disables macrophages and lymphocytes, the same monocytic immune cells that control TB pathogenesis. New *M. tuberculosis* infections in people already immunocompromised by HIV infection can progress rapidly to disease. The mechanism of monocytic dysfunction, nevertheless, remains unknown. In vitro studies by Meylan et al. failed to demonstrate differences in phagocytosis or intracellular mycobacterial growth between HIV-infected and HIV-uninfected macrophages. They also failed to demonstrate an effect of mycobacterial infection on HIV replication, as measured by the release of p24 antigen from macrophage supernatants.[58] Most[44,51–53,60,63] but not all other investigators[57,64] also failed to detect abnormal cytokine gene expression in HIV-infected macrophages. Meylan et al. conclude that the enhanced mycobacterial growth seen in HIV-infected people cannot be explained by a direct cellular effect of HIV on macrophages. Possible mechanisms of HIV-induced susceptibility to mycobacteria include deficient T-cell or natural killer cell activity, or an indirect in vivo effect of HIV causing phagocyte dysfunction independent of phagocyte infection.[58]

Whatever the mechanism, DTH is impaired in HIV-infected people. The HIV-induced loss of CD4-bearing lymphocytes is associated with an inability to mount cutaneous DTH responses to antigens, such as tuberculin purified protein derivative (PPD), mumps, trichophyton, *Candida,* and tetanus toxoid.[3] Anergy, the absence of cutaneous DTH, is well known to characterize an advanced stage of HIV disease[74] and to predict the occurrence of AIDS-defining conditions.[3] Impaired DTH also diminishes the usefulness of the tuberculin skin test. For this reason, in 1990 the American Thoracic Society and the CDC recommended that the definition of a positive tuberculin skin test (using 5 tuberculin units [TU] of intradermal PPD) in HIV-infected people be changed from the previous value of ≥ 10 mm of induration to a value of ≥ 5 mm of induration.[15] Nevertheless, many persons coinfected with both HIV and *M. tuberculosis* are anergic to tuberculin[56] and are at high risk for active TB.[61,79]

RISK OF TUBERCULOSIS IN HIV-INFECTED PERSONS

HIV-infected people are more likely to develop active disease from newly acquired *M. tuberculosis* infection than people who do not have HIV. These uninfected people have an approximate 30% risk of becoming infected with *M. tuberculosis* after a close household exposure[4] and, once infected with *M. tuberculosis,* face an approximate 3% risk of active TB in the first year and lower risks thereafter.[31,75] The higher risks conferred by HIV infection have been alarmingly demonstrated by analyses of institutional TB outbreaks in recent years.[6,17–19,22,33,35–37] DiPerri et al. documented the rapid progression of newly acquired TB in HIV-infected hospitalized patients. Among 18 patients with negative tuberculin skin tests who were exposed to patients hospitalized with active TB, eight developed active TB, seven within 60 days of exposure. The mean CD4 lymphocyte count was lower in patients who developed TB than in those who did not.[35] Daley et al. described an investigation of a TB outbreak in a congregate-living facility for HIV-infected people. Using restriction fragment length polymorphism (RFLP), a method of DNA fingerprinting, to identify the *M. tuberculosis* strain of the index active case, they confirmed transmission of the strain to 11 (37%) of 30 exposed people within 106 days. One patient developed active disease 4 weeks after exposure. Another 4 (13%) of the 30 patients developed positive tuberculin skin tests.[33] Dooley et al. described a nosocomial TB outbreak in a hospital unit for HIV-infected patients in Puerto Rico. Eight (17%) of 48 exposed people developed active TB (35.7 cases per 100 person-years), with a median incubation period of 80 days.[36] The high risk of disease is also demonstrated by a retrospective cohort study of HIV-infected patients in Spain. Among 10 nonanergic patients who converted from negative to positive tuberculin skin tests, three patients subsequently developed TB. Three of 36 anergic patients also tuberculin converted, and TB developed in two of them.[61]

The HIV-associated accelerated onset of TB was even more alarmingly demonstrated in institutional outbreaks of multidrug-resistant TB (MDR-TB). In 1991 the CDC described MDR-TB outbreaks in four hospitals in Miami and New York involving 147 patients. Eighty-three patients had AIDS, indicating advanced immunodeficiency. The case-fatality rate was extremely high due to the combination of immunodeficiency, drug resistance, and delayed diagnosis. Eight cases of TB were reported in health care workers, four of whom were HIV-infected. One HIV-infected health care worker died from MDR-TB.[22] In the Miami outbreak, MDR-TB, as opposed to drug-sensitive TB, was associated with previous hospitalization on the HIV ward, the use of aerosolized pentamidine and intravenous treatments in the HIV clinic, and the diagnosis of AIDS.[17,40] In one of the New York hospital outbreaks, MDR-TB was also associated with HIV infection and with low CD4 lymphocyte cell counts.[71] In another of the New York outbreaks, RFLP analysis confirmed the spread of the same strain within an AIDS inpatient ward. The attack rate for all exposed patients was 6.1%, and the rate was 9.5% for exposed patients located two rooms away or closer to the patient with the active case. TB was diagnosed 1–3.5 months after exposure to the infectious case.[37] Drug-resistant tubercle bacilli are thought to be transmitted in the same manner as drug-susceptible bacilli. Infection rates among contacts of active TB patients, furthermore, are similar for both drug-resistant and drug-susceptible organisms.[27] However, active cases of MDR-TB are more likely to be infectious for longer periods of time.[17,27]

The high risk of exogenous TB infection in HIV-infected patients has even resulted in exogenous reinfection. Using RFLP analysis, Small et al. documented how five HIV-infected patients with drug-sensitive TB became exogenously reinfected with new MDR-TB strains. Six other patients in their study also developed MDR-TB but did not change their RFLP pattern, indicating that drug resistance developed in their original stains.[82] Exogenous reinfection was considered uncommon prior to the AIDS epidemic, presumably because of the immunity conferred by the initial infection. Most cases of MDR-TB, however, are thought to be initial infections with resistant strains or the development of drug resistance in an initially drug-sensitive strain. The extent of exogenous reinfection in HIV-infected patients and its role in the growth of MDR-TB are still unknown.

HIV-infected people with latent *M. tuberculosis* infection have a high risk of reactivation disease. People without HIV but with positive tuberculin skin tests for more than 7 years have a TB reactivation risk of approximately 0.07–0.1 cases per 100 patient-years.[31,32,75] Selwyn et al. documented the far higher rate in HIV infection among intravenous drug users in a methadone-maintenance treatment program in The Bronx, New York. Over a mean follow-up of 22 months, 7 (14%) of 49 HIV-infected, tuberculin positive ($\geq$ 10 mm of reactivity) people developed

TB (7.9 cases per 100 patient-years) but none of 62 tuberculin-positive people without HIV infection developed TB.[77] In another 31-month prospective study with a similar population, they found that 4 (16%) of 25 HIV-infected tuberculin positive (≥ 5 mm of reactivity) patients developed TB (9.7 cases per 100 patient-years) and five (7%) of 68 HIV-infected anergic patients developed TB (6.6 cases per 100 patient-years), but only 1 (2%) of 59 tuberculin-positive (≥ 10 mm of reactivity) patients without HIV developed TB (1.0 cases per 100 patient-years).[79] Similar results were found by Moreno et al., who studied only HIV-infected persons in Madrid, with a median follow-up of 26 months: 24 (28%) of 84 tuberculin-positive (≥ 5 mm of reactivity) patients developed TB (10.4 cases per 100 patient-years); 19 of 151 (13%) nonanergic, tuberculin-negative people developed TB (5.4 cases per 100 patient-years); and 20 of 112 (18%) anergic people developed TB (12.4 cases per 100 patient-years).[61] These studies suggest that the TB reactivation risk in HIV-infected patients is approximately 100 times greater than patients not infected with HIV.

CLINICAL MANIFESTATIONS OF TB AMONG HIV-INFECTED PERSONS

M. tuberculosis is relatively more virulent than most opportunistic pathogens of AIDS. *Pneumocystis carinii* pneumonia characteristically does not occur in HIV-infected people until the CD4 count falls below 200 cells/mm^3, and *Mycobacterium avium* complex disease usually does not occur until the CD4 count falls below 100 cells/mm^3. However, TB is found in HIV-infected patients with a wide range of immune function, from very low to normal CD4 counts, with a median of about 300–400 cells/mm^3.[87] The greater virulence of *M. tuberculosis* in HIV-infected patients often results in active TB preceding other opportunistic infections. Approximately half of the cases of TB precede, a tenth are concurrent with, and the remainder follow other AIDS-defining conditions.[28,59,81,85] The reader should be aware of an element of confusion in terminology caused by the changing surveillance definition of AIDS. Originally TB was not an AIDS-defining condition. The CDC revised the AIDS case definition in 1987 to include extrapulmonary TB in HIV-infected people[11] and again in 1993 to include any manifestations of TB in HIV-infected patients.

TB in HIV-infected patients with no or mild immunodeficiency often presents with "typical" clinical manifestations. In moderate-to-severe immunodeficiency, three "atypical" features of TB are usually found: cutaneous anergy, "atypical" pulmonary manifestations, and high rates of extrapulmonary disease. These distinctions have not been fully documented, because most case series with immunological data are small. Other than these distinctions, TB in HIV-infected patients at any stage of immunodeficiency usually presents with constitutional symptoms (fever, malaise, weight loss, night sweats, chills) and often with respiratory symptoms (cough, sputum production) that are common in many other HIV-related conditions.

Cutaneous anergy, induced by HIV-associated immunodeficiency, is found not only in patients with latent *M. tuberculosis* infection but also in patients with active disease. In a San Francisco study of TB patients, 61% of patients with AIDS and 9% of patients without AIDS had non-significant tuberculin skin test responses (< 10 mm induration).[28] Similar findings were found among TB patients in another San Francisco study (20% of HIV-infected vs. 7% of uninfected patients were anergic)[87] and in a study in Zaire (33% vs. 7%).[30]

Pulmonary manifestations, reflected in chest radiograph findings, range from upper-lobe disease with cavities in patients with no or mild immunodeficiency, to lower-lobe disease, miliary patterns, an absence of cavities, intrathoracic adenopathy, and occasionally normal chest radiographs in patients with moderate-to-severe immunodeficiency.[28,30,35,38,39,45,59,73,85–87] In severely immunocompromised patients, cavitation is uncommon and adenopathy is found frequently.[38,45,54,72,73] Adenopathy is an uncommon finding in immunocompetent adults with TB.[45]

High rates of extrapulmonary TB, 45–79%, are characteristic of HIV-infected patients.[9,10,34,73] In a report of TB among AIDS patients in Newark, New Jersey, between 1981 and 1985, 21 of 29 (79%) patients had extrapulmonary disease, in contrast to the extrapulmonary rate of 27% among all TB patients in Newark and 16% among all TB patients in the United States in 1984.[85] Extrapulmonary disease has been found in 60% of AIDS/TB patients in San Francisco[28,81] and 50% in New York City.[54] In an HIV-seroprevalence study of 3,077 patients in 20 TB clinics nationwide, HIV infections were more frequent in patients with extrapulmonary TB (19.8%) and both extrapulmonary and pulmonary disease (15.6%) than in patients with pulmonary disease alone (10.2%).[68] Overall, HIV-infected patients were twice as likely to have extrapulmonary disease than were uninfected patients.[68] Similarly, in Zaire more patients with extrapulmonary disease were HIV-seropositive (45%) than patients with pulmonary TB (33%).[30] Among HIV-infected patients, furthermore, patients with extrapulmonary disease are likely to have lower CD4 counts than people without extrapulmonary disease.[87]

Extrapulmonary disease in HIV-infected patients commonly occurs in the lymphatic system, gastrointestinal and genitourinary tracts, or the bone marrow.[28,54,59,72,87] Disseminated disease is also common, reportedly occurring in approximately half of patients.[73,87] Central nervous system TB has appeared in approximately 3–10% of patients in AIDS/TB series.[2,28,78,85] *M. tuberculosis* bacteremia, uncommon in patients not infected with HIV, is not unusual.[28,59,77] Tuberculous pericarditis,[34,85] peritonitis,[78] and rectal abscess,[85] and scrotal TB have also been reported.[86]

Diagnosis of TB in HIV-infected patients requires a higher index of clinical suspicion because of the high likelihood of tuberculin skin test anergy, "atypical" pulmonary manifestations, and extrapulmonary disease. Chest radiographs may be nonspecific and not suggestive of TB. Acid-fast smear and culture of available clinical specimens, including respiratory secretions, bronchial washings, lung tissue, pleural fluid, lymph node tissue, bone marrow, blood, urine, stool, brain biopsy, and cerebrospinal fluid, are essential elements of the investigation. Sputum smears in HIV-infected patients have similar[82,87] or slightly lower sensitivity[34,49]—approximately 50–60%[38,81,87]—than smears in uninfected TB patients, though higher in another series.[59] Bronchoscopic biopsy and/or bronchoalveolar lavage fluid smear, culture, and pathology add to the sensitivity of sputum analysis.[84] Despite the increased risk of cutaneous anergy in HIV infection, tuberculin skin testing is often helpful in diagnosis. Approximately 70% of HIV-infected patients without an AIDS-defining condition and approximately 30% of AIDS patients will respond to 5 TU PPD with $\geq$ 10 mm of induration.[1]

Delayed diagnosis of TB, made more likely by several decades of decreasing incidence and physicians' lack of familiarity with the clinical manifestations of TB in HIV-infected patients, poses a hazard for health care workers and their patients. Flora et al. describe a series of 11 patients for whom the diagnosis of TB was not suspected. Even in patients with "typical" manifestations of TB, many of the appropriate diagnostic tests were not performed. *P. carinii* pneumonia was the presumed diagnosis in nine of these patients but was confirmed in only one.[42] The index case in the hospital outbreak described by DiPerri et al. had a cough but a normal chest radiograph; antituberculous therapy was not begun until the 28th day of hospitalization because of the low index of suspicion of TB.[35] In the MDR-TB outbreak in four hospitals in New York and Miami, the TB diagnosis was delayed because chest radiographs did not show "typical" TB patterns.[22]

PREVENTION OF TB AMONG HIV-INFECTED PERSONS

HIV-infected persons should be routinely screened for tuberculous infection with the tuberculin skin test. The CDC recommends that $\geq$ 5 mm induration 48–72 hours after 5 TU intradermal PPD be the criterion for a positive test in HIV-infected people and people with risk factors for HIV infection whose HIV infection status is unknown but who are suspected of being infected.[14] Patients with a positive test and pulmonary disease should be promptly examined and tested for active TB. Those without evidence of active TB most likely have latent infection and are at high risk for active infection in the near future. Such people should be considered for preventive therapy with isoniazid (300 mg daily for one year).[15]

Several studies support preventive therapy with isoniazid in HIV-infected tuberculin reactors. In two studies of HIV-infected tuberculin reactors in a methadone maintenance program in The Bronx, the TB incidence rate was 7.9 and 9.7 cases per 100 person-years among those who did not take preventive therapy, but zero among those who took preventive therapy.[78,79] A similar study mostly of intravenous drug users with positive tuberculin tests was conducted in Madrid. After 22 months of observation TB occurred in 29 (31%) of 94 patients who did not take isoniazid and in one (3.7%) of 27 patients who took isoniazid.[61] In an unpublished study in Zambia in HIV-infected patients (unstated tuberculin status), 6 months of preventive therapy with isoniazid reduced the subsequent TB rate over an average of a half year of observation from 4.4% to none.[89] These observations were recently confirmed in a clinical trial conducted among HIV-infected people in Haiti. Over approximately 3 years, active TB occurred in 2 (5%) of 38 tuberculin-positive patients who received a 12-month course of isoniazid plus vitamin B6 (1.7 cases per 100 person-years) but in 6 (24%) of 25 patients who received vitamin B6 alone (10.0 cases per 100 person-years). Remarkably, preventive therapy with isoniazid was also found to delay progression to HIV disease, AIDS, and death.[69]

HIV-infected people should also be tested for cutaneous anergy.[21] Several decision analyses have concluded that the benefits of isoniazid preventive therapy outweigh the risks for anergic HIV-infected people who live in communities with high prevalences of TB.[48,76] A clinical study is ongoing to test this practice. The CDC recommends that preventive therapy with isoniazid should be considered for anergic people who are known contacts of infectious TB patients and who are from groups in which the prevalence of tuberculous infection is at least 10%.[21]

The CDC has also recently issued preventive therapy guidelines for HIV-infected and uninfected people who have been exposed to an active case of MDR-TB. Included in the guidelines are recommended methods to estimate the likelihood of new infection with *M. tuberculosis* and with MDR-TB and considerations for preventive therapy decision making.[24]

Occupational settings raise several important issues of TB prevention.[16] Workers with risk factors for having HIV infection should be offered voluntary HIV testing following counseling.[13] Workers with positive tuberculin skin tests and with immunosuppressing medical conditions, including HIV infection, are at higher risk than those without HIV for reactivation TB.[61,78,79] Such people should be counseled about taking preventive therapy with isoniazid.[15] Workers with immunosuppressing medical conditions, including HIV infection, are also at higher risk for newly acquired TB disease. For this reason, infection control administrative measures and engineering controls are even more important for immunosuppressed workers than for healthy workers.[16] The best protection for severely immunodeficient workers is to avoid exposure to patients with active TB. Therefore, severely immunodeficient workers should have the option available of voluntary transfer to areas with the lowest risk. These issues, also discussed in other chapters, highlight the importance of worker education, voluntary interventions, effective infection control programs, and counseling workers to make informed personal decisions.

TREATMENT OF TB AMONG HIV-INFECTED PERSONS

The principles of initial TB treatment are the same regardless of whether the patient is infected with HIV: to promptly initiate effective multidrug antituberculosis therapy based on clinical and drug-resistance surveillance data. All hospitalized patients with potentially infectious TB should be promptly placed in respiratory isolation rooms with negative pressure relative to adjacent areas. In the author's hospital, which serves a population with a high prevalence of TB, all HIV-infected patients with even a low index of suspicion of active pulmonary TB are placed in respiratory isolation rooms.

Because of the increasing incidence of multidrug-resistant TB in the United States, the CDC recently issued updated recommendations for the treatment of TB. These recommendations include the need for in vitro drug susceptibility testing of *M. tuberculosis* isolates from all patients and reporting of these results to the health department, initial four-drug regimens for the treatment of TB, and directly observed therapy for patients with TB.[27] In several series, antituberculosis therapy appeared to be as effective regardless of the patient's HIV status.[28,73,81] Because data from controlled clinical trials are not available to determine if 6-month regimens are adequate for HIV-infected patients with TB, the CDC recommends that such patients be treated for a total of 9 months and for at least 6 months after sputum conversion.[13,27]

CONCLUSIONS

The impact of HIV infection on TB morbidity and mortality globally and in the United States is enormous. TB is one of the most common opportunistic infections in people with HIV infection. In many developing and industrialized nations, the number of reported cases of TB is increasing. The association between the immunodeficiency induced by HIV infection and the increase in TB morbidity and mortality is becoming clearer. As a result, the World Health Organization and the CDC have issued guidelines on the need for preventive therapy for *M. tuberculosis* infection and for prompt diagnosis and adequate treatment of TB both in people who are infected and not infected with HIV.[13,14,21,24,27,47] The atypical presentation of TB in HIV-infected patients makes delayed diagnosis more likely, increasing the risk for other patients and for health care workers. In 1990 the CDC issued guidelines, which will be revised in the near future, for preventing the spread of TB in health care settings.[16] Outbreaks in residential and health care institutions since then underscore the need for rigorous adherence to infection control procedures.

REFERENCES

1. Barnes PF, Bloch AB, Davidson PT, Snider DE: Tuberculosis in patients with human immunodeficiency virus infection. N Engl J Med 324:1644–1650, 1991.
2. Berenguer J, Moreno S, Laguna F: Tuberculous meningitis in patients infected with human immunodeficiency virus. N Engl J Med 326:668–762, 1992.
3. Blatt SP, Hendrix CW, Butzin CA, et al: Delayed-type hypersensitivity skin testing predicts progression to AIDS in HIV-infected patients. Ann Intern Med 119:177–184, 1993.
4. Bloch AB, Reider HL, Kelly GD, et al: The epidemiology of tuberculosis in the United States. Semin Respir Infect 4:157–170, 1989.
5. Bloom BR, Murray CL: Tuberculosis: Commentary on a reemergent killer. Science 257:1055–1064, 1992.
6. Braun MM, Coté TR, Rabkin CS: Trends in death with tuberculosis during the AIDS era. JAMA 269:2865–2868, 1993.
7. Braun MM, Truman BI, Maguire B, et al: Increasing incidence of tuberculosis in a prison inmate population: Association with HIV infection. JAMA 261:393–397, 1989.
8. Brudney K, Dobkin J: Reemergent tuberculosis in New York City: Human immunodeficiency virus, homelessness, and the decline of tuberculosis control programs. Am Rev Respir Dis 144:745–749, 1991.
9. Centers for Disease Control: Tuberculosis and acquired immunodeficiency syndrome—Florida. MMWR 35:587–590, 1986.
10. Centers for Disease Control: Tuberculosis and acquired immunodeficiency syndrome—New York City. MMWR 36:785–795, 1987.
11. Centers for Disease Control: Revision of the CDC surveillance case definition of acquired immunodeficiency syndrome. MMWR 36(suppl 1):3S–15S, 1987.
12. Centers for Disease Control: A strategic plan for the elimination of tuberculosis in the United States. MMWR 38(SS-3):1–25, 1989.
13. Centers for Disease Control: Tuberculosis and human immunodeficiency virus infection: Recommendations of the Advisory Committee for the Elimination of Tuberculosis (ACET). MMWR 38:236–238, 243–250, 1989.
14. Centers for Disease Control: Screening for tuberculosis and tuberculous infection in high-risk populations: Recommendations of the Advisory Committee for the Elimination of Tuberculosis. MMWR 39(RR-8):1–7, 1990.
15. Centers for Disease Control: The use of preventive therapy for tuberculous infection in the United States: Recommendations of the Advisory Committee for the Elimination of Tuberculosis. MMWR 39(RR-8):9–12, 1990.
16. Centers for Disease Control: Guidelines for preventing the transmission of tuberculosis in health care settings, with special focus on HIV-related issues. MMWR 39(RR-17):1–29, 1990.
17. Centers for Disease Control: Nosocomial transmission of multidrug-resistant tuberculosis to health care workers and HIV-infected patients in a urban hospital—Florida. MMWR 39:718–722, 1990.
18. Centers for Disease Control: Tuberculosis among residents of shelters for the homeless—Ohio, 1990. MMWR 40:869–877, 1991.
19. Centers for Disease Control: Tuberculosis outbreak among persons in a residential facility for HIV-infected persons—San Francisco. MMWR 40:649–652, 1991.
20. Centers for Disease Control: Tuberculosis morbidity in the United States: Final data. MMWR 40(SS-3):23–27, 1991.
21. Centers for Disease Control: Purified protein derivative (PPD)-tuberculin anergy and HIV infection: Guidelines for anergy testing and management of anergic persons at risk of tuberculosis. MMWR 40:27–33, 1991.
22. Centers for Disease Control: Nosocomial transmission of multidrug-resistant tuberculosis among HIV-infected persons—Florida and New York. MMWR 40:585–591, 1991.
23. Centers for Disease Control: The HIV/AIDS epidemic: The first 10 years. MMWR 40:357–369, 1991.
24. Centers for Disease Control: Management of persons exposed to multidrug-resistant tuberculosis. MMWR 41(RR-11):59–71, 1992.
25. Centers for Disease Control: Tuberculosis morbidity—United States, 1992. MMWR 42:363, 1993.
26. Centers for Disease Control and Prevention: HIV/AIDS Surveillance Report 5(1):4–5, 1993.
27. Centers for Disease Control and Prevention: Initial therapy for tuberculosis in the era of multidrug resistance: Recommendations of the Advisory Council for the Elimination of Tuberculosis. MMWR 42(RR-7), 1993.

28. Chaisson RE, Schecter GF, Theuer CP, et al: Tuberculosis in patients with the acquired immunodeficiency syndrome: Clinical features, response to therapy, and survival. Am Rev Respir Dis 136:570–574, 1987.
29. Chaisson RE, Slutkin G: Tuberculosis and human immunodeficiency virus infection. J Infect Dis 159:96–100, 1989.
30. Colebunders RL, Ryder RW, Nzilambi A, et al: HIV infection in patients with tuberculosis in Kinshasa, Zaire. Am Rev Respir Dis 139:1082–1085, 1989.
31. Comstock GW, Livesay VT, Woolpert SF: The prognosis of a positive tuberculin reaction in childhood and adolescence. Am J Epidemiol 124:1–16, 1974.
32. Comstock GW: Prevention of tuberculosis among tuberculin reactors: Maximizing benefits, minimizing risks. JAMA 256:2729–2730, 1986.
33. Daley CL, Small PM, Schecter GF, et al: An outbreak of tuberculosis with accelerated progression among persons infected with the human immunodeficiency virus. An analysis using restriction-fragment length polymorphisms. N Engl J Med 326:231–235, 1992.
34. D'Cruz IA, Sengupta EE, Abrahams C, et al: Cardiac involvement, including tuberculous pericardial effusion, complicating acquired immunodeficiency syndrome. Am Heart J 112:1100–1102, 1986.
35. Di Perri G, Cruciani M, Danzi MC, et al: Nosocomial epidemic of active tuberculosis among HIV-infected patients. Lancet 2:1502–1504, 1989.
36. Dooley SW, Villarino ME, Lawrence M: Nosocomial transmission of tuberculosis in a hospital unit for HIV-infected patients. JAMA 267:2632–2635, 1992.
37. Edlin BR, Tokars JI, Grieco MH, et al: An outbreak of multidrug-resistant tuberculosis among hospitalized patients with the acquired immunodeficiency syndrome. N Engl J Med 326:1514–1521, 1992.
38. Elliott AM, Luo M, Tembo G, et al: Impact of HIV on tuberculosis in Zambia: A cross sectional study. BMJ 301:412–415, 1990.
39. Eriki PP, Okwera A, Aisu T, et al: The influence of human immunodeficiency virus infection on tuberculosis in Kampala, Uganda. Am Rev Respir Dis 143:185–187, 1991.
40. Fischl MA, Daikos GL, Uttamchandani RB, et al: Clinical presentation and outcome of patients with HIV infection and tuberculosis caused by multiple-drug-resistant bacilli. Ann Intern Med 117:184–190, 1992.
41. Fischl MA, Uttamchandani RB, Daikos GL, et al: An outbreak of tuberculosis caused by multiple-drug-resistant tubercle bacilli among patients with HIV infection. Ann Intern Med 117:177–183, 1992.
42. Flora GS, Modilevsky T, Antoniskis D, Barnes PF: Undiagnosed tuberculosis in patients with human immunodeficiency virus infection. Chest 98:1056–1059, 1990.
43. Frieden TR, Sterling T, Pablos-Mendez A, et al: The emergence of drug-resistant tuberculosis in New York City. N Engl J Med 328:521–526, 1993.
44. Gendelman HE, Friedman RM, Joe S, et al: A selective defect on interferon α production in human immunodeficiency virus-infected monocytes. J Exp Med 172:1433–1442, 1990.
45. Hopewell PC: Impact of human immunodeficiency virus infection on the epidemiology, clinical features, management, and control of tuberculosis. Clin Infect Dis 15:540–547, 1992.
46. [Reference deleted.]
47. Joint WHO/IUATLD Working Group on HIV Infection and Tuberculosis: Tuberculosis and AIDS. Bull Int Union Against Tuberc Lung Dis 64:8–11, 1989.
48. Jordan TJ, Lewitt EM, Montgomery RL, Reichman LB: Isoniazid as preventive therapy in HIV-infected intravenous drug abusers: A decision analysis. JAMA 265:2987–2991, 1991.
49. Klein NC, Duncanson FP, Leonx TX III, et al: Use of mycobacterial smears in the diagnosis of pulmonary tuberculosis in AIDS/ARC patients. Chest 95:1190–1192, 1989.
50. Kochi A: The global tuberculosis situation and the new control strategy of the World Health Organization. Tubercle 72:1–6, 1991.
51. Kornbluth RS, McCutchen JA: Skin test responses as predictors of tuberculous infection and progression of HIV-infected persons. Ann Intern Med 119:242–243, 1993.
52. Kornbluth RS, Munis JR, Oh PS, et al: Characterization of a macrophage-tropic HIV strain that does not alter macrophage cytokine production yet protects macrophages from superinfection by vesicular stomatitis virus. AIDS Res Hum Retroviruses 6:1023–1026, 1990.
53. Locksley RM, Crowe S, Sadick MD, et al: Release of interleukin 1 inhibitory activity (contra IL-1) by human monocyte derived macrophages infected with human immunodeficiency virus in vitro and in vivo. J Clin Invest 82:2097–2105, 1988.
54. Louie E, Rice LB, Holzman RS: Tuberculosis in non-Haitian patients with acquired immunodeficiency syndrome. Chest 90:542–545, 1986.

55. Mann JM, Welles SL: Global aspects of the HIV epidemic. In DeVita VT, Hellman S, Rosenberg SA (eds): AIDS: Etiology, Diagnosis, Treatment, and Prevention. 3rd ed. Philadelphia, JB Lippincott, 1992, pp 89–98.
56. Markowitz N, Hansen NI, Wilcosky TC, et al: Tuberculin and anergy testing in HIV-seropositive and HIV-seronegative persons. Ann Intern Med 119:185–193, 1993.
57. Merrill JE, Koyanagi Y, Chen ISY: Interleukin-1 and tumor necrosis factor alpha can be induced from mononuclear phagocytes by human immunodeficiency virus type 1 binding to the CD4 receptor. J Virol 63:4404–4408, 1989.
58. Meylan PRA, Munis JR, Richman DD, Kornbluth RS: Concurrent human immunodeficiency virus and mycobacterial infection of macrophages in vitro does not reveal any reciprocal effect. J Infect Dis 165:80–86, 1992.
59. Modilevsky T, Sattler FR, Barnes PF: Mycobacterial disease in patients with human immunodeficiency virus infection. Arch Intern Med 149:2201–2205, 1989.
60. Molina JM, Schindler R, Ferriani R, et al: Production of cytokines by peripheral blood monocytes/macrophages infected with human immunodeficiency virus type 1 (HIV-1). J Infect Dis 161:888–893, 1990.
61. Moreno S, Baraia-Etxaburu J, Bouza E, et al: Risk for developing tuberculosis among anergic patients infected with HIV. Ann Intern Med 119:194–198, 1993.
62. Murray JF. The white plague: Down and out, or up and coming? Am Rev Respir Dis 140:1788–1795, 1989.
63. Munis JR, Richman DD, Kornbluth RS, et al: HIV-1 infection of macrophages in vitro neither induces TNF/cachexin gene expression nor alters TNF/cachexin induction by lipopolysaccharide. J Clin Invest 85:591–596, 1992.
64. Nakajima K, Martínez-Maza O, Hirano T, et al: Induction of IL-6 (B cell stimulatory factor-2/IFN-β2) production by HIV. J Immunol 142:531–536, 1989.
65. Nolan CM, Elarth AM, Barr HA, et al: An outbreak of tuberculosis in a shelter for homeless men: A description of its evolution and control. Am Rev Respir Dis 143:257–261, 1991.
66. Nolan CM, Heckbert S, Elarth A: Case-control study of the association between immunodeficiency virus infection and tuberculosis [abstract]. Program and abstracts of the Fourth International Conference on AIDS, Washington, DC, 1988.
67. [Reference deleted.]
68. Onorato IM, McCray E: Prevalence of human immunodeficiency virus infection among patients attending tuberculosis clinics in the United States. J Infect Dis 165:87–92, 1992.
69. Pape JW, Jean SS, Ho JL, et al: Effect of isoniazid prophylaxis on incidence of active tuberculosis and progression of HIV infection. Lancet 342:268–272, 1993.
70. Pape JW, Liautaud B, Thomas F, et al: Characteristics of the acquired immunodeficiency syndrome (AIDS) in Haiti. N Engl J Med 309:945–950, 1983.
71. Pearson ML, Jereb JA, Frieden TR, et al: Nosocomial transmission of multidrug-resistant Mycobacterium tuberculosis: A risk to patients and health care workers. Ann Intern Med 117:191–196, 1992.
72. Pitchenik AE, Burr J, Suarez M, et al: Human T-cell lymphotropic virus-III (HTLV-III) seropositivity and related disease among 71 consecutive patients in whom tuberculosis was diagnosed. Am Rev Respir Dis 135:875–879, 1987.
73. Pitchenik AE, Cole C, Russell BW, et al: Tuberculosis, atypical mycobacteriosis, and the acquired immunodeficiency syndrome among Haitian and non-Haitian patients in south Florida. Ann Intern Med 101:654–655, 1984.
74. Redfield RR, Wright DC, Tramont EC: The Walter Reed staging classification for HTLV III/LAV infection. N Engl J Med 314:131–132, 1986.
75. Reider HL, Cauthen GM, Comstock GW, Snider DE: Epidemiology of tuberculosis in the United States. Epidemiol Rev 11:79–98, 1989.
76. Rose DN, Schechter CB, Sacks HS: Preventive medicine for HIV-infected patients: An analysis of isoniazid prophylaxis for tuberculin reactors and for anergic patients. J Gen Intern Med 7:589–594, 1992.
77. Saltzman BR, Motyl MR, Friedland GH, et al: Mycobacterium tuberculosis bacteremia in the acquired immunodeficiency syndrome. JAMA 256:390–391, 1986.
78. Selwyn PA, Hartel D, Lewis A, et al: A prospective study of the risk of tuberculosis among intravenous drug users with human immunodeficiency virus infection. N Engl J Med 320:545–550, 1989.
79. Selwyn PA, Sckell BM, Alcabes P: High risk of active tuberculosis in HIV-infected drug users with cutaneous anergy. JAMA 268:504–509, 1992.
80. Slutkin G, Leowski J, Mann J: The effects of the AIDS epidemic on the tuberculosis problem and tuberculosis programmes. Bull Int Union Tuberc Lung Dis 63:21–24, 1988.

81. Small PM, Schecter FG, Goodman PC, et al: Treatment of tuberculosis in patients with advanced human immunodeficiency virus infection. N Engl J Med 324:289–294, 1991.
82. Small PM, Shafer RW, Hopewell PC: Exogenous reinfection with multidrug-resistant Mycobacterium tuberculosis in patients with advanced HIV infection. N Engl J Med 328:1137–1144, 1993.
83. Snider DE, Hutton MD: Tuberculosis in correctional institutions. JAMA 261:436–437, 1989.
84. So SY, Lam WK, Yu DYC: Rapid diagnosis of suspected pulmonary tuberculosis by fiberoptic bronchoscopy. Tubercle 63:195–200, 1982.
85. Sunderam G, McDonald RJ, Maniatis T, et al: Tuberculosis as a manifestation of the acquired immunodeficiency syndrome (AIDS). JAMA 256:362–366, 1986.
86. Sunderman G, Mnagura BT, Lombardo JM, Reichman LB: Failure of "optimal" four-drug short-course tuberculosis chemotherapy in a compliant patient with human immunodeficiency virus. Am Rev Respir Dis 136:1475–1478, 1987.
87. Theuer CP, Hopewell PC, Elias D, et al: Human immunodeficiency virus infection in tuberculosis patients. J Infect Dis 162:8–12, 1990.
88. Tuberculosis, New York City: City Health Information, New York City Department of Health, March 1991.
89. Wadhawan D, Hira S, Mwansa N, et al: Isoniazide prophylaxis among patients with HIV-1 infection. Program and abstracts of the Sixth International Conference on AIDS, San Francisco, June 19–23, 1990.

STEVEN B. MARKOWITZ, MD

EPIDEMIOLOGY OF TUBERCULOSIS AMONG HEALTH CARE WORKERS

From the Division of Environmental and Occupational Medicine
Mount Sinai School of Medicine
New York, New York

Reprint requests to:
Steven B. Markowitz, MD
Division of Environmental and Occupational Medicine
Box 1057
Mount Sinai School of Medicine
1 Gustave L. Levy Place
New York, NY 10029

The reversal of the decline of tuberculosis in the United States beginning in the 1980s has ignited a high level of concern among health care workers during the past few years. This concern is due principally to three factors: the overall increase in the incidence of tuberculosis, its relative ease of transmission, and the rise of multidrug-resistant organisms. The increased incidence of tuberculosis raises a number of issues. First, the resurgence of the disease undermines the conviction that the march of progress against diseases, especially infectious diseases, is irreversible. Second, unlike HIV infection, tuberculosis is acquired through inhalation, a route of transmission that would be considered "casual contact" in a world with HIV infection. Third, the specter of untreatable tuberculosis causes alarm, especially among the younger and middle-age workers who have no memory of a time when medicines effective against tuberculosis were not available. Finally, since tuberculosis has led to untold numbers of human deaths over the centuries and continues to cause a large number worldwide, ancient fears about the disease probably continue to be transmitted culturally to recent generations.

The specific occupational relevance of recent changes in the incidence, age distribution, and other risk factors for tuberculosis is important. First, if the overall incidence of tuberculosis is an important factor in determining the numbers and types of workers at risk for occupationally acquired TB, occupational studies conducted in the late 1970s and early 1980s would be relevant, since the national rate of tuberculosis in the early 1990s matches that of the late 1970s. At the same time, the concentration of tuberculosis among people with specific risk factors such as HIV infection, homelessness, and imprisonment has the occupational consequence that workers in industries that serve people with these risk factors will have the highest risk of exposure to tuberculosis. Secondly, the increase in TB since 1985 has mostly occurred in 25- to 44-year-olds,[13] which is the group most likely to be working. Their presence in workplaces while in the early stage of tuberculosis may lead to exposure to TB among coworkers in a wide variety of workplaces. Third, since as much as 25% of cases of tuberculosis occur among foreign-born individuals,[13] especially recent immigrants, workplaces employing such individuals may present a higher likelihood of tuberculosis transmission than other workplaces, especially if the workplace is crowded and poorly ventilated. The employment of large numbers of Asian and Caribbean immigrants in garment sweatshops in New York City is an example of such workplaces.

While not a focus of this volume, it is important to remember that some occupations involve exposure to silica, a situation in which an increase in the risk of developing active tuberculosis is well documented.[32,41,46,50] There is still significant exposure to silica in the United States and elsewhere.[26,50] If the incidence of tuberculosis continues to rise and spreads beyond populations with specific risk factors, workers exposed to silica will have increased exposure to tuberculosis with a predictable outcome.

A RISK MODEL OF TB TRANSMISSION

One of the principal advantages of epidemiology is the insight that it can provide into constructing an appropriate model of causation and transmission of disease. The risk factors measured in epidemiologic studies are variably useful proxies for the elements of such a model. Given the lack of technical feasibility of measuring the concentration of *Mycobacterium tuberculosis* (Mtb) organisms in the air, epidemiologic measures of the components of risk become more important. It is nonetheless useful to describe a prevailing model of tuberculosis transmission in order to have a framework by which to judge the utility of the epidemiologic findings reviewed in the following sections.

The risk of acquiring TB infection depends principally upon the dose of tubercle bacilli received and possibly on host factors. As with any external toxin, the dose of tubercle bacilli to a worker depends upon the concentration of organisms in the worker's breathing space, the volume of infection-laden air inhaled by the susceptible worker, and the duration of exposure to the relevant concentration.[16] The concentration of organisms in the breathing space depends on the balance between the introduction of organisms into the air by tuberculosis patients and the elimination or dilution of such organisms. The introduction of viable organisms into the air is a function of how many infectious bacilli are in the sputum and the propensity of the organisms to become airborne by coughing, sneezing or recruitment of organisms through special procedures such as sputum induction, administration of aerosolized medicines, bronchoscopy, or by the use of a saw during autopsy. Elimination or dilution of such expelled mycobacterial organisms is influenced by building ventilation, alterations in the size of the space in which organisms are released, and the presence of ultraviolet radiation. On the other side of the balance, the volume of infection-laden air inhaled by the susceptible worker is a product of the pulmonary ventilation (breathing volume per unit time) multiplied by the duration of exposure to the infection-laden air.

Riley and others have formalized these relationships into a model for airborne transmission of infection.[47,48] The model is based in part on the work of Wells in the 1950s and 1960s, which designates the dose of *M. tuberculosis* organisms (1 or more) necessary to produce an infection as a *quantum*.[53] The number of *M. tuberculosis* organisms needed to produce an infection is unknown. The model of Riley and others asserts the following:[47,48]

$$N = \text{concentration} \times \text{volume} = Iq/Q \times Spt = S(Iqpt/Q)$$

where N = number of quanta inhaled by susceptibles
I = number of infectors (patients with active TB)
q = rate of production of quanta per infector
Q = volume of fresh air in which quanta are distributed
S = number of susceptibles
p = pulmonary ventilation per susceptible
t = duration of exposure

One of the assumptions of such a model is that the *M. tuberculosis* organisms are evenly distributed in the air into which they are released so that the dose of organisms that susceptible workers receive depends solely upon the volume of air that they breathe. Since the distribution of infectious organisms in the air is more likely to be random than even, Riley and colleagues modified their model to assign a Poisson distribution to describe the likelihood of infection, so that

$$C, \text{ or number of new infections} = S(1-e^{-Iqpt/Q})$$

The probability of infection becomes $(1-e^{-Iqpt/Q})$.[47,48]

This model has most often been used empirically in outbreak investigations.[10,38,47] Such investigations usually yield I, S, C and Q and allow reasonable estimations of p and t. The variable q, the rate of production of quanta per infector, is obtained, and the infectiousness of the index case in the outbreak can be characterized. By this method, a study by Catanzaro obtained a q of 249 units per hour produced by a TB patient who underwent intubation and bronchoscopy,[10] and a study by Nardell obtained a q of 13 units per hour in a TB patient who was infecting coworkers in an office setting.[38] The considerable range of q's obtained from different studies suggests that TB patients vary greatly in their degree of infectiousness. An alternative explanation is that the model does not fully or correctly capture the variables determining risk of infection.

At a clinical level, important factors that affect the available dose are the clinical presentation (presence of cavitary disease in the lungs), the presence of viable organisms on sputum smear, delay in proper diagnosis, delay in instituting effective treatment, and premature cessation of treatment. Multidrug-resistant TB organisms are not known to be more infectious per se but may lead to higher occupational exposures through atypical clinical presentation and delays in proper diagnosis and treatment. Available and accessible health care for people at high risk of TB is an obvious *sine qua non* for the proper clinical care of patients with tuberculosis.

The risk of acquiring TB infection may also depend upon unidentified host factors. Usually, fewer than a third of close contacts of patients with active TB become infected. While this may be due to differences in doses received by the contacts or to a random process, the existence of host factors, immunologic or otherwise, that enhance or reduce the likelihood of infection is plausible. If they exist, they have not been identified.

LIMITATIONS OF CURRENT EPIDEMIOLOGIC STUDIES

While the existence of excess risk of acquiring TB under certain conditions in health care settings is undisputed, the level of this excess risk and the relative importance of conditions of exposure leading to this risk are less certain. Much of the uncertainty derives from methodologic limitations that are common to many of the epidemiologic studies published in recent decades concerning the occupational risk of TB. Errors of measurement of exposure and outcome significantly undermine the ability of such studies to characterize the risk of occupational TB. Proper comparison populations from the community at large are usually lacking, making it difficult to define the level of risk that is attributable to occupational exposure. Sample size is often limited, especially in outbreak investigations, leading to difficulty in evaluating the level of risk associated with specific jobs, job tasks, duration of exposure, and interactions of these factors.

Given the inability to measure directly the airborne concentration of *M. tuberculosis,* characterization of potential exposure to Mtb is necessarily crude. At best, some studies, usually the outbreak investigations, report duration of potential exposure, job title and tasks, type of interaction with infectious patients, and number of infectious patients.[10,24,28,29] Quantification of these variables, when applicable, is usually limited. Job titles and responsibilities vary among studies, making comparisons across studies difficult. Description of environmental controls such as type and rate of ventilation, presence of isolation rooms, work practices, and availability and use of respirators, all of which would modify the exposure to Mtb organisms, is often ignored or reported descriptively. Studies of the incidence of PPD conversion among large groups of hospital workers usually derive from routine surveillance activities of employees health services and frequently include no measures of potential exposure except the number of admissions for TB and the general area or department where tested employees work.[6,7,49] Dilution of the population at risk by large numbers of workers with no occupational contact with tuberculosis patients will result in predictably low rates of PPD conversion. Such inattention to and variation in exposure measurement severely limits the ability to interpret, much less compare, the PPD conversion rates yielded by many of the studies to date.

More universally acknowledged are the limitations of the PPD skin test and its use among occupational groups as a measure of infection. Proper use of the test requires careful attention to appropriate storage and application of the test material and interpretation of the resultant skin reaction. Rates of false positive and false negative tests due to cross-reactivity and anergy, respectively, may be significant and can be expected to vary across studies depending on the geographic location, age distribution, and other characteristics of the study populations. Measures to limit the rate of false positivity, including two-step testing to detect a booster response[10,30] and screening with an anergy panel, are rarely used in published studies. Detection of the timing of infection requires serial testing and still leaves unanswered exactly when infection occurred during the interval between tests.

For all of the limitations of the PPD test as an accurate technic, the most serious problem with its use in epidemiologic studies is the lack of compliance with a periodic testing schedule, as recommended by the CDC.[12] Most studies rely to varying degree upon the skin testing results provided by routine PPD surveillance programs undertaken by the employees' health service. Few research studies have specifically included longitudinal PPD testing of health care workers. In outbreak investigations, PPD surveillance performed by employees' health services often provides the pre-exposure PPD status, although some studies have used PPD tests applied immediately after exposure as a measure of baseline infection status. Broader incidence studies rely wholly upon routine surveillance PPD testing to obtain time-specific PPD conversion rates. To the extent that all employees are not tested on a regular basis, the time of potential exposure to TB will vary among the study population. For incidence studies, such variation limits the ability to use annual PPD conversion rates as a measure of infection, since it is not clear when the PPD conversions occurred. For outbreak investigations, lack of frequent and periodic testing increases the uncertainty that infection occurred as a specific result of the outbreak being studied. The lack of resources provided to hospital employees' health services to perform routine PPD testing and incomplete participation of employees in PPD testing programs have had the unintended but serious result of limiting the ability to study the risk of TB infection among health care workers.

The issue of how much the health care worker's risk of acquiring TB is determined by community or household exposure versus occupational exposure has received little scientific attention in recent years. This is due in part to the low rate of TB in the general population and in part to the presumption of work-relatedness of TB occurring in health care workers, as reflected by the recent policy guidelines issued by OSHA.[40] Some studies refer to the crude PPD conversion rates in the surrounding community or the general population[1,3,6] in interpreting PPD conversion rates observed among workers in hospitals. Such comparisons ignore the known variation of PPD positivity rates by age, gender, socioeconomic class, and community.[46] Measuring community exposure by PPD testing of household contacts or by asking PPD converters and controls about home or neighborhood exposure to tuberculosis have been little used as methods of separating the contribution of different sources of risk of infection for the health care worker. Even if used, though, these methods might present problems of incomplete testing and accuracy of recall.

OUTBREAK INVESTIGATIONS

Outbreak investigations describing occupational acquisition of tuberculosis from a single index patient or well-defined set of patients have been vital in drawing attention to the occupational consequences of the reemergence of TB in the past decade. Such investigations have demonstrated the magnitude of risk in different settings, usually under conditions of suboptimal environmental and infection controls. To a lesser extent, studies of nosocomial outbreaks have also elucidated the components of the risk of exposure to TB for health care workers. Major limitations of outbreak investigations have included the frequent absence of baseline PPD test results, the difficulty of extrapolating the results of such investigations to nonoutbreak conditions of TB exposure, and, frequently, small sample sizes preventing detailed analyses. Table 1 lists most of the recently published outbreak investigations as well as some classic studies from previous decades. Most, but not all, of these studies will be reviewed in this chapter.

In 1972, Ehrenkranz and Kicklighter[24] described a contact investigation of health care workers exposed to a patient whose TB was not diagnosed until

TABLE 1. Outbreak Investigations

Authors (year)	Setting/Patients	Risk of TB in HCWs	Status of Infection and Environmental Controls
Ehrenkranz & Kick-lighter (1972)	Hospital Miami 1 index case intubated 5-day hospital stay	24/100 (24%) PPD conversions 11/19 (58%) PPD conversions among HCWs with close contact 10/41 (24%) PPD conversions among HCWs with little or unknown contact	Poor ventilation documented Isolation room under positive presure Contaminated air recirculated onto ward
Catanzaro (1982)	Hospital intensive care unit San Diego 1 index case (smear-negative TB) 7-day hospital stay	14/45 (31%) PPD conversions 10/13 (77%) PPD conversions among HCWs present at bronchoscopy	Poor ventilation No report on respirators used
Lundgren et al. (1987)	Hospital autopsy rooms Sweden 2 patients died with undiagnosed TB	4 HCWs attending autopsies developed active TB	Environmental conditions not reported
Kantor et al. (1988)	VA hospital Chicago (medical ward, autopsy room) 1 index case undiagnosed until histology exam of autopsy tissue	9/56 (16%) PPD conversions among exposed HCWs versus 3/333 (1%) conversions unexposed HCWs RR = 17.8 3 HCWs developed active TB	No mechanical ventilation on medical ward: no isolation Autopsy room had 11 air changes/hour and no air recirculation
Haley et al. (1989)	Hospital emergency department (ED) Dallas 1 index case with known cavitary TB 5-hour stay in ED	16/62 (26%) PPD conversions among ED workers 12/26 (46%) PPD conversions among ED workers who worked the same shift as the index case 6 HCWs developed active TB disease	Recirculated air without filtration Surgical masks used
Hutton et al. (1990)	Rural hospital Arkansas 1 index case with draining TB abscess	33/45 (73%) PPD conversions among HCWs who worked on patient's floor 26/29 (90%) PPD conversions among HCWs who entered patient's room > 10 times	Abscess was drained and irrigated with aerosol generating appliance Isolation room was under positive pressure in relation to hallway Recirculated air with no reported filtration
MMWR (1991)	Substance abuse treatment residence Michigan 1 MDR TB case with HIV	15/69 (22%) contacts (clients and staff) converted PPDs	No controls in place
Pearson et al. (1992)	Hospital New York City MDR TB in 23 HIV-infected patients	11/32 (34%) PPD conversions in TB-exposed workers versus 1/47 (2%) PPD conversions in TB nonexposed workers	Patient rooms had positive pressure Patients allowed to wander without masks
Beck-Sague et al. (1992)	Hospital Miami MDR TB in HIV-infected patients on HIV ward and clinic during 2-year study period	13/39 (33%) PPD conversions on HIV ward and clinic vs. 0/15 (0%) PPD conversions on thoracic surgery service	Some rooms had positive pressure Inadequate triage of patients with suspected TB Delay in use of isolation; early discharge from isolation
Pierce et al. (1992)	Hospital, hospice (medical ward) Texas 1 index case with AIDS, *P. carinii* and MAC Diagnosis of TB delayed for 5 months	19/93 (20%) HCWs in hospital converted 11/65 (17%) HCWs in hospice converted 1 active TB case	Environmental conditions not reported

autopsy. The index case was admitted for pulmonary edema, intubated in the emergency department, and was on assisted ventilation until his death 5 days later. The patient spent 2½ days (57 hours) on a medical floor before being transferred to an intensive care unit on a different floor, where he stayed for 3 days (67 hours). Throughout his hospital stay, he produced large amounts of sputum and underwent frequent nasotracheal sectioning. A total of 24 TB skin test conversions occurred among 100 employees (24%) who worked in the three areas of the hospital where the index case was treated. In subgroup analysis, there were 11 skin test conversions among 19 workers (58%) who directly cared for the patient while he was on the medical floor. In addition, 10 of 41 workers (24%) on the medical floor who only briefly entered the patient's room or who had no known contact with the patient also experienced PPD conversions.

PPD conversions were also analyzed by occupational title. Ten of the 23 (43%) physicians and medical students who had contact with the index case had a skin test conversion, including 7 of 10 (70%) who had close contact with the patient. Among other job titles, 9 of 54 (17%) nurses and nursing aides and 2 of 8 (25%) ward secretaries also developed positive PPD skin tests.

Environmental controls, especially on the medical floor, were deficient. Central air conditioning with 70% recycled air provided ventilation for the medical floor, mixing air from the patient rooms and the working areas of the floor. Air in the index patient's room was under positive pressure with respect to the corridors. The ventilation system contained no high-efficiency filters.

This study had several important findings. It showed that when sufficient numbers of infectious particles are generated, even for a brief relative period of time (57 hours), the majority of people exposed may become infected. Secondly, under such conditions, a significant percentage of people who may have little or no known direct contact with the patient but who worked in the general vicinity where the patient is treated may acquire TB infection. Finally, the significant difference between infection rates among health care workers on the medicine floor (21/60, or 35%) and intensive care unit (2/19, or 11%), shows that even modest differences in environmental conditions in the same facility may have a significant impact on the infection rate produced by highly infectious patients.

Catanzaro[10] reported a very high PPD conversion rate among health care workers due to airborne transmission from a patient whose sputum was repeatedly negative for tubercle bacilli. An alcoholic with chronic obstructive pulmonary disease was admitted for 5 days to a university hospital where he was on assisted ventilation for 3 days and underwent bronchoscopy for 2½ hours. Ten of the 13 (77%) health care workers who were present at bronchoscopy had PPD conversions. Fourteen of 45 (31%) health care workers who had contact with this patient developed newly positive PPD skin tests. Attendance at bronchoscopy was highly related to PPD conversion. In addition, the rate of PPD conversion increased with the number of hours that workers were exposed to the index case. Of note, the ventilation was grossly inadequate in the bronchoscopy room (1.2 air exchanges per hour). No ultraviolet lights were present in the facility, and no comments were made on the use of the personal respiratory protection. Catanzaro concluded that sputum-smear negative cases of tuberculosis may under certain conditions be as infectious as smear-smear positive cases of tuberculosis.

In 1989, Haley et al.[28] documented an unusual outbreak of active tuberculosis among emergency department workers at a large public hospital in Dallas. A 70-year-old alcoholic with known cavitary tuberculosis was admitted to the emergency department for 4 hours before being transferred to the medical intensive care unit. While in the emergency department, he underwent intubation with placement on a ventilator. He was described as producing large amounts of sputum that obstructed the orotracheal tube. Sixteen of the 62 (26%) tuberculin-negative employees who worked in the emergency department on the day the index case was present subsequently converted their skin test. Among employees who worked on the same shift as when the patient was treated, 12 of 26 (46%) developed a newly positive PPD skin test within 5 months after exposure, compared to 4 of 36 (11%) emergency department employees who worked other shifts on the same day. Six emergency department employees developed active tuberculosis during the year following exposure to the index case. Some of these cases of active disease were believed to derive from exposure to one of the other employees who had developed TB subsequent to exposure to the index case (worker-to-worker transmission). The isolates from four of the emergency department nurses with active TB were similar with respect to susceptibility patterns and phage typing, suggesting a common source of disease.

The environmental controls in place in this emergency department were inadequate. The air-handling unit in the emergency department recycled 60% of the air without adequate filtration. Surgical masks were the only respiratory protection available.

In summary, this study demonstrates a high PPD conversion rate following a short but intense employee exposure to tubercle bacilli. The setting was a known case of cavitary tuberculosis treated in an area with grossly inadequate environmental controls and personal protective equipment. The extraordinarily high rate of active TB disease that developed among exposed workers was not fully explained.

Hutton et al.[29] investigated a highly unusual episode of infectivity associated with manipulation of draining TB abscess in 1990. A 67-year-old man with a history of gastrectomy and prolonged corticosteroid therapy was admitted with left hip pain. A CT scan demonstrated a thigh abscess, and the patient was taken to the operating room, where surgical incision, drainage, and irrigation were performed. For the following 3 days, a large amount of drainage was reported from the abscess area. Beginning on the third post-surgical day and extending throughout the remainder of the patient's hospitalization, the abscess cavity was irrigated with an aerosol-generating appliance. The patient worsened and was transferred to the intensive care unit on the sixth postoperative day. After 3 days, he returned to the medical floor and died 5 days later. Twenty-eight of 33 (85%) hospital employees with exposure to the index case on the medical floor during the week following surgery converted their PPD skin test; 26 of 29 (90%) of workers who reported entering the patient's room more than 10 times during the week following surgery developed positive PPDs. In a larger group of employees who reported working at least 1 day on the medical floor where the patient was located during the week following surgery, 33 of 45 (73%) developed newly positive PPD skin tests.

The investigators also documented the infection experience of the patients and visitors who spent some time on the medical floor where the index case was treated. Prevalences of positive PPD tests were reported, since serial PPD testing was not feasible. Ten of 22 patients (45%) who stayed in the room across from the room of the index case or spent time in the outpatient recovery room, which was 40 feet from the room of the index case, showed positive PPD tests, compared to 2 of 29 (7%) patients who stayed in rooms that were at least 100 feet from the room of the index case. Among patients and visitors who spent 1 day or less in the outpatient recovery room during the first 3 days of use of the irrigation appliance, 9 of 37 (24%) showed a positive PPD skin test compared to 5 of 63 (8%) of patients and visitors who visited the similar amount of time in the same recovery room during the final 9 days of the index case's hospitalization, subsequent to the peak aerosolization of abscess material. The relative risk of positive PPD status was 3.1 (95% CI = 1.1–8.5). Finally, nine cases of active tuberculosis were associated with this outbreak, affecting five hospital employees, two patients, and two members of the index case's family who visited him in the hospital.

In 1991, the Centers for Disease Control published evidence of occupational acquisition of tuberculosis from four hospital outbreaks involving patient-to-patient transmission of multidrug-resistant tuberculosis.[14] In this report, three New York City hospitals and one Miami hospital reported a total of 130 cases of multidrug-resistant tuberculosis between 1989–1991. Most of the patients had HIV infection, and most (80%) died within 1 to 4 months of diagnosis of TB. The CDC report demonstrated nosocomial acquisition of multidrug-resistant TB for many of these patients.

As part of these nosocomial outbreaks, eight health care workers at the four hospitals developed active tuberculosis. The overall population at risk was not determined. Notably, five of six of the health care workers whose HIV status was known were HIV-positive. Furthermore, in at least some of these health care workers, the tubercle bacilli isolated from their sputum showed a genetically identical pattern to the patients for whom they cared, demonstrating that the TB was acquired from the patients.

Additional detail from one of these outbreaks was provided by Beck-Sague et al.,[5] who studied occupational acquisition of tuberculosis among workers exposed to patients with tuberculosis on a HIV ward and clinic at Jackson Memorial Hospital in Miami. From March 1988 to April 1990, 13 documented PPD conversions occurred among 39 workers (33%) on the HIV ward and clinic. This was significantly higher (p = .01) than the 0 of 15 skin test conversions among health care workers employed on the thoracic surgery service, where TB patients were rarely hospitalized. For the 10 employees who worked on the HIV ward and whose PPD skin test converted, there was a strong correlation between their risk of *M. tuberculosis* infection during a given month and the number of days that sputum smear-positive patients with multidrug-resistant TB were hospitalized on the HIV ward ($r = 0.75$, $p = 0.005$). No significant correlation was found between the workers' risk of infection and the number of days that sputum smear-positive patients with drug-susceptible TB were hospitalized.

Enforcement of infection control procedures and environmental controls were inadequate. Some patients were not initially placed in isolation, and others were removed from isolation rooms while they were still infectious. The doors of isolation rooms were sometimes left open, and the occupants of the isolation rooms sometimes left their rooms without consistently wearing their masks. Not all isolation rooms were under negative pressure. In the HIV clinic, there was no procedure for segregating patients who might have tuberculosis, and the rooms where aerosolized pentamidine was administered were adjacent to a larger treatment room. Improved control measures were instituted after recognition of the problem of nosocomial TB infection among patients and staff.

In 1992, Pearson et al. at the CDC published a report on occupational TB exposure relating to a nosocomial outbreak of multidrug-resistant TB among mostly HIV-infected patients at a large New York City hospital.[42] Twenty-three multidrug-resistant TB patients and 48 drug-susceptible TB patients were hospitalized during the 18-month study period. Documented PPD conversions during the study period were associated with exposure to TB: 11 of 32 (34%) health care workers working on the AIDS unit or the medical floor converted the PPD versus 1 of 47 health care workers (2%) assigned to other areas of the hospital ($p < 0.001$). Half of the health care workers (6/12) assigned to the AIDS unit acquired TB infection during the study period.

TB transmission in a different type of health care setting, a substance abuse treatment facility, was reported in Michigan in 1991.[15] The index case was a HIV-positive intravenous drug user who had been treated in a different state for tuberculosis with three drugs and who then moved to Michigan, where he entered a substance abuse treatment facility. He continued to have pulmonary symptoms and reported to the county TB clinic, where a sputum positive for Mtb was obtained. Sputum culture later showed multidrug-resistant organisms. Serial PPD testing of 69 residents and staff in the facility who initially had tuberculin negative skin tests showed a documented skin test conversion in 15 (22%). An additional 16 people (11%) of the 140 people originally tested had positive PPD skin tests at initial testing and may have been infected by the index case.

SURVEILLANCE STUDIES

Incidence and prevalence studies of tuberculosis infection in health care workers allow a more systematic evaluation of the risk of TB infection than the outbreak investigations in two ways. First, these studies potentially better reflect the risk of TB experienced by health care workers under "usual," (nonepidemic) conditions of exposure. Secondly, this second group of studies should better reflect the risk of TB among a larger group of workers. Table 2 shows the relevant studies published during the past 15 years describing the annual rate of skin test conversion among different groups of workers. The annual PPD skin test conversion rate among hospital workers in most of the studies listed in Table 2 dating from the late 1960s to the mid-1980s was 1–2%. Many of the hospitals studied admitted relatively few patients with tuberculosis during the time period studied. Furthermore, many studies report PPD conversion rates for all workers or job titles in the hospitals under study. Such studies often include large groups of hospital workers with little or no exposure to patients with tuberculosis.

By contrast, the more recent studies generally show higher rates of conversion than the studies cited above.[17,23,25,33,34,35] These latter studies report the PPD experience of smaller groups of workers than the earlier studies—that is, the workers with significant exposure to patients with tuberculosis. The most informative studies listed in Table 2 are reviewed below.

In one of the few studies of active tuberculosis, Ashley and Wigle evaluated the incidence of active disease among hospital employees in Ontario, Canada, from 1966 to 1969.[2] They found 164 cases, of which two thirds (110) occurred among nurses and student nurses. Physicians in training had the highest rate of active tuberculosis (81 per 100,000 per year, based on five cases), followed by radiology and laboratory technicians (60 per 100,000) and nurses of various categories (18 to 55 per 100,000). Dietary, clerical, and miscellaneous personnel had the lowest rate of tuberculosis (16 per 100,000 per year). Only a minority of cases (23/164, 14%) occurred among recent PPD converters. The remainder were considered by the authors to be a result of previous infection, that is, from the

TABLE 2. Surveillance Studies

Author	Setting (No. of TB Patients)	Study Period	Population	Incidence/Comments
Barrett-Connor (1979)	California medical schools	mid 1960s–mid 1970s	medical students	1–2% PPD conversion rate/year
Atuk & Hunt (1971)	University hospital, Virginia	1968–1969 (2 years)	hospital workers (n = 1,253)	1.9% PPD conversion rate/year (all hospital employees) 6.6% PPD conversion rate/year (workers with close contact with patients) 2 active cases among HCW
Gregg & Gibson (1975)	State TB hospital, South Carolina	1969–1973 (5 years)	hospital workers (n = 449)	16.2% PPD conversion rate/ 5 years 25% PPD conversion/5 years among HCWs with direct patient contact 2 active TB cases
Berman et al. (1981)	Community hospital, Baltimore (58 TB patients)	1971–1976	hospital workers (n = 1900)	1.4% PPD conversion rate/year Highest rates in laundry, maintenance and housekeeping
Craven et al. (1975)	University hospital, Virginia (17 cases of unsuspected TB: refers active TB cases elsewhere)	1972–1973 (15 months)	hospital workers (n ≈ 2,500)	1.7% PPD conversion rate/ 15 months among HCWs with contact with unsuspected TB cases 0.25% PPD conversion rate/ 15 months in HCWs without such contact
Vogeler & Burke (1978)	University-affiliated hospital, Salt Lake City (9 TB cases/year)	1972–1976 (5 years)	hospital workers (n = 6,335)	0.1% PPD conversion rate/ 5 years 1% PPD conversion rate/5 years among HCWs in TB contact investigations
Ruben et al. (1977)	University-affiliated hospital, Pittsburgh (25 TB cases/year)	1973–1975 (2.5 years)	hospital workers (n = 626)	7.7% PPD conversion rate/ 2.5 years Conversion rate not increased in workers with direct contact with patients
Dandoy & Hanson (1975)	11 hospitals in Arizona	1973–1975 (2 years)	hospital workers (n = 8,066)	3.5% PPD conversions (time period unspecified)
Bryan & McVicker (1977)	Community hospital, Columbia, SC (24 TB patients)	1976 (6 months)	hospital workers (number unspecified)	4.5% PPD conversion rate/ 6 months
Chan & Tabak (1985)	Urban public hospital, Miami	1977–1981	house staff physicians (n = 221)	4% PPD conversion/year Increased cumulative conversion rates with increased years of employment 2 active TB cases
Capewell et al. (1988)	National Health Service employees in Lothian region of Scotland (900 TB patients)	1978–1984	health care workers (n ≈ 22,000)	15 cases of active TB among HCWs (only pathology technicians showed increased incidence)
Price et al. (1987)	156 hospitals, North Carolina	1980–1984	hospital workers (n = 71,253)	1.14% PPD conversions/year
	Same hospitals	1983–1984	hospital workers	active TB case rate: ~ 9/100,000 in HCWs ~ 13/100,000 in general population
Aitken et al. (1987)	64 hospitals, Washington state (787 TB patients)	1982–1984 (3 years)	hospital workers (n ≈ 51,000)	0.1% PPD conversion rate/ 3 years

(Continued on following page)

TABLE 2. Surveillance Studies *(Continued)*

Author	Setting (No. of TB Patients)	Study Period	Population	Incidence/Comments
Raad et al. (1989)	University hospital (UH) (4 TB cases/year)	1984–1987	hospital workers (UH: n ≈ 3,100)	0.13% PPD conversions/year at UH
	vs. psychiatric hospital (PH) (1 TB case/year) Florida	1985–1987	(PH: n ≈ 3,100)	0.42% PPD conversions/year at PH
Malasky et al. (1990)	14 urban hospitals in U.S.	mid 1980s (3 years)	physicians in training in pulmonary medicine and infectious diseases (n = 104)	11% PPD conversions/3 years among pulmonary fellows versus 2.4% PPD conversions/3 years among infectious disease fellows
Calder et al (1989)	Public primary care clinic, Florida	1987–1988	clinic staff members (n = 76)	17/72 (24%) staff converted in 18 months 13 HCWs had positive prevalent PPDs Odds ratio = 15 for being in room when aerosolized pentamidine was administered Inadequate air exchange No HEPA filter Positive pressure treatment room
Edlin et al. (1992)	Hospital, New York City MDR-TB in 118 HIV-infected patients	1989	hospital workers	18% conversions in 16 months (numbers not provided) 1 active MDR-TB case in HCW with RFLP pattern matching patient Isolation rooms had positive pressure
Dooley et al. (1992)	Hospital, Puerto Rico TB in HIV-infected patients	1989–1990	hospital workers (n = 908)	Prevalence study: 54/109 (50%) nurses exposed to TB patients had positive PPDs vs 35/188 (19%) positive PPDs among clerical workers with no TB exposure ($p = 0.0005$) Isolation rooms had positive pressure Recirculated air was not filtered
Fagan & Poland (1994)	U.S. medical schools	early 1990s	medical students (101 U.S. medical schools, number of students not available)	Estimated 1.8% mean annual PPD conversion rate among medical students 15/75 (20%) schools reported ≥ 4% PPD conversion rate for their medical students
Boudreau (NIOSH) (1992–1994)	Urban public hospital, Miami	1989–1992	hospital workers (n = 607)	6% annual PPD conversion rate among 263 exposed HCWs vs. 0.6% among 344 unexposed workers Adjusted RR = 11.9 Incomplete isolation facilities Improper application of isolation procedures

period prior to the hospital employment in Ontario. The authors concluded that much of the active TB among the hospital workers that they studied was the result of long-term infection and not the result of occupational acquisition during the time studied.

In the early 1970s, Craven et al. prospectively evaluated the PPD experience of 2,500 employees at a general hospital where all patients with active tuberculosis were referred to a nearby sanatorium.[18] Hence, employees in this hospital only had exposure to 17 initially unsuspected cases of tuberculosis between mid 1972 and mid 1973. The average time between admission and isolation for suspected tuberculosis was 5 days. Once properly diagnosed, patients were transferred to the sanatorium. Among personnel who were exposed to patients with tuberculosis, 8 of 484 (1.65%) converted the PPD skin test versus 5 of 2,013 (0.25%) of unexposed health care workers. The sixfold increase in PPD conversion rate among the exposed employees was highly statistically significant ($p = 0.0003$). The PPD conversion rate was highest among workers with contact with the five patients whose chest x-ray findings were typical of tuberculosis but were overlooked by the treating physicians. Workers who were most likely to have exposure to unsuspected cases of tuberculosis were x-ray technicians and licensed practical nurses. Overall, the conversion rates are low in this study compared to other studies, but they are of interest because the study isolates the risk of unsuspected tuberculosis for hospital workers.

In 1974–1975, Barrett-Connor surveyed 4,140 physicians from California medical schools to describe their personal histories of latent and active tuberculosis.[4] Among physicians who graduated from medical school in the decade after World War II, 194 of 644 (30%) reported PPD conversion during medical school. An additional 106 of the remaining 450 (24%) reported having a skin test conversion during the subsequent 20–30 years of their medical careers. Thus, more than half of the occupational risk of TB infection for physicians between ages 46–55 was acquired during medical school. This disproportionate risk of TB infection during the medical school years continued among physicians graduating from medical school between 1956 and 1975, but at lower levels. Among physicians who gave a history of active tuberculosis, ages 21 to 35 were the most frequent years of developing active disease. This is not surprising given the increased period of developing active disease experienced by recent PPD converters. Among physicians graduating from 1966–1975, only 40 of 669 (6%) reported PPD conversion during medical school, which translates to a 1–2% annualized conversion rate. Despite this dramatic decrease in tuberculosis infection among medical students and during their subsequent medical careers, Barrett-Connor noted that the prevalence of PPD positivity among physicians remained twice the rate for the U.S. population.

Capewell et al.[9] in Britain reported 15 new cases of pulmonary tuberculosis among 22,000 National Health Service workers from 1978–1983 in a region of Scotland. Average annual incidence is 11 per 100,000 for all workers. Only one occupational group, medical laboratory technicians, had a significantly higher rate, 111 cases per 100,000 per year, which was based on only two cases. The overall rate of TB among National Health Service workers was lower than that of working age adults in the surrounding geographic area and in Scotland as a whole.

Chan and Tabak studied the PPD conversion rate among housestaff at Jackson Memorial Hospital, a public hospital in Miami, in the late 1970s and early 1980s.[17] Miami had the highest rate of tuberculosis among major United States cities during this time: Jackson Memorial Hospital had 247 admissions for TB in 1981. Study results were based on self-reported conversions among house staff. The authors found a 4% annualized PPD conversion rate for house staff among all specialties and all four training years. The proportion of house staff reporting PPD conversions increased with added years of training, reflecting a longer period of exposure. First-year residents (PGY 1s) showed 2% skin test conversions, which the authors consider to be low as a result of incomplete retesting. By comparison, the percentage house staff reporting PPD conversions was 8.6% for PGY 2s, 11% for PGY 3s, and 14.3% for PGY 4s. These percent conversions for residents above PGY 1 refer to cumulative rates reflecting all years of training. Both the nature and the magnitude of the trend toward increasing conversions with increasing duration of house staff employment suggests that the acquisition of tuberculosis was occupational. Two cases of active tuberculosis were diagnosed among house staff physicans whose PPD skin test converted during training.

Malasky et al.[37] surveyed the PPD conversion experience of pulmonary and infectious disease physicians at 14 urban training programs in the U.S. in 1983. Seven of 62 (11%) pulmonary fellows reported skin test conversions during their two-year training program versus just 1 of 42 (2.4%) infectious disease fellows.

Calder et al. studied transmission of TB to workers at a publicly funded primary care clinic in Florida.[8,11] Seventeen of 72 (24%) staff members developed positive PPD tests in the 18-month study period. An additional 13 workers had a positive PPD when first tested. In a case-control analysis to examine risk factors for PPD conversion, being in the room when aerosolized pentamidine was administered was associated with an OR of 15 (95% CI = 1.4–730). Other significant risk factors included working on the floor where TB patients were treated (OR = 9.3; 95% CI = 1.1–420) and being nonwhite (OR = 7.9; 95% CI = 1.4–79). Clinical areas of the building received less than six air exchanges per hour. All but 90% of the air supply for the clinical area was recycled after passing through large particle filters only. The treatment room where aerosolized pentamidine was administered was under positive pressure with respect to the hallways.

DiPerri et al. in Italy studied active tuberculosis among health care workers at five inpatient health care facilities where tuberculosis was treated between 1986–1991.[20,21] Because health care workers receive bacille Calmette-Guérin vaccine in Italy, no analysis by PPD conversion rate was possible. The investigators compared the frequency of active tuberculosis among nurses at three inpatient units where 85 HIV-infected patients were treated for tuberculosis to nurses at two inpatient facilities where 1,079 patients not infected with HIV were treated for tuberculosis during the six years of the study. Seven of 135 (5.2%) nurses working at the HIV units versus 2 of 106 (1.9%) nurses who worked in the non-HIV facilities developed active tuberculosis. The authors obtain a relative risk of 44.4 (95% CI = 8.5–438) when comparing the number of cases of active TB among nurses per year per 100 hospitalized patients for the two types of units (8.2/year/100 patients at the HIV units vs. 0.19/year/100 patients at the non-HIV units). No description of infection control procedures and environmental controls is provided aside from the assertion that "facial masks are worn routinely." The authors concluded that the patients with HIV and tuberculosis may disseminate TB more readily than tuberculosis patients without HIV. Limitations of the study include the failure to address possible differential HIV infection rates among nurses at the two types of facilities and the lack of details regarding duration of employment and intensity of contact that nurses had with patients at the two types of units.

Dooley et al. studied the prevalence of positive PPDs among health care workers at a large public hospital with a special HIV unit in Puerto Rico.[22] Patients with TB were admitted to the HIV unit and to the internal medicine service. Since baseline PPD testing had not been routinely done, analysis of conversions were not possible. Two thirds (908/1,420) of the health care workers in the hospital were interviewed and skin tested. Clerical workers on floors of the hospital where TB was not treated formed the reference group. (The percentage rates reported in this paragraph were adjusted for age and history of community TB exposure.) Their rate of positive PPDs was 35 of 188 (17%). By comparison, 9 of 19 (56%) nurses in the HIV unit had positive PPDs (OR = 6.4; 95% CI = 2.2–18). Among nurses on the internal medicine wards, 45 of 90 (55%) had positive PPDs (OR = 6.0; 95% CI = 3.3–11). Nurses from other services, where TB was not treated, had a rate of positive PPD similar to that of the clerical workers, 44/224 (19%), yielding an OR = 1.2 (95% CI = 0.7–2.0). Interestingly, among the group of ancillary workers, which included escorts, housekeepers, and maintenance workers, 48/114, (39%) had positive PPDs (OR = 3.1, 95% CI = 1.8–5.4). It was not specified whether these workers worked in areas of the hospital where TB patients were treated.

Two additional findings of this study are interesting. A reported history of community exposure to TB increased the risk of having a positive skin test (OR = 2.5; 95% CI = 1.5–2.4), but the magnitude of the increased risk was less than that associated with working with TB patients. Also, the authors noted that the environmental controls at the hospital were poor. Rooms on the HIV ward and the isolation rooms on the internal medicine service were under positive pressure with respect to the corridor. Recirculated air was not filtered. Also, many of the patients with TB were not admitted to isolation rooms.

Fagan and Poland have published a 1992 survey of U.S. medical schools to assess the risk of PPD conversions among medical students throughout the United States.[25] They obtained questionnaire data from 101 of 126 (80%) medical schools. Fewer than half of the schools surveyed required PPD testing on an annual basis. For the 75 schools reporting PPD conversion rates, the mean conversion rate was 1.8%, and the median was 2%. Fifteen of the 75 schools (20%) reported annual PPD conversion rates of 4% or higher, with the highest being 12%. No breakdown by year of medical school was provided.

Investigators from NIOSH have conducted the most specific recent surveillance study designed to characterize the risk of TB infection among hospital workers. A full description of the 4-year study had not been published as of October 1994, but preliminary communications provide useful information.[33-35] Boudreau and others reviewed the PPD testing program of selected employees at Jackson Memorial Hospital from 1989–1992. This is the same Miami hospital where a multidrug-resistant TB outbreak was documented in 1989–1991[5] and where Chan and Tabak described a 4% annual conversion rate among house staff in the early 1980s.[17] Boudreau et al. defined exposed workers as those working on four internal medicine inpatient wards, the medical intensive care unit, and the emergency department. A comparison group was drawn from employees in areas of the hospital where patients with TB were reportedly not treated. The exposed workers underwent PPD testing approximately every 4 months, and the unexposed group were PPD tested approximately every 12 months during the 4-year study period.

Data from the first 3 years of the study are available.[33–35] Among 263 exposed workers (contributing 551 person-years at risk), 33 had skin test conversions during the 3-year study period, yielding a 6% annual conversion rate. By contrast, among the 344 unexposed workers (with 866 person-years at risk), there were 5 PPD skin test conversions, yielding a 0.6% annual conversion rate. The relative risk adjusted for age, ethnicity, and gender was 11.9 (95% CI = 4.6–30.7).[34] Analysis by job title showed that ward clerks had the highest PPD conversion rate, 17% (5 of 29), during the study period, followed by nurses with a 14% PPD conversion rate (21 of 155).[33] The rate of conversion among exposed workers was much higher in the first 2 years of the study period (6.2% in 1989, 7.1% in 1990) than in the third study year (2.7% in 1991).[34]

Administrative and environmental controls to prevent TB were clearly suboptimal for at least the first 2 years of the study. These are described in part in the summary of Beck-Sague's study[5] in the preceding section. Proper isolation facilities were not available, and appropriate isolation procedures were not followed. Improvements in these controls made in 1991 were believed to be partly responsible for the decline in the PPD conversion rate among exposed workers in 1991 and 1992.[33–35]

This NIOSH study is important for several reasons. The exposed group was defined more broadly than in most recent surveillance and outbreak studies. Participants were followed for a long time, PPD testing was frequent, job titles were recorded, and risk by job title was analyzed. Changes in environmental controls were recorded.

Interestingly, the PPD conversion rate among exposed workers in the NIOSH study was as high as any of the rates obtained in other surveillance studies, including those by Chan and Tabak,[17] Malasky et al.,[37] and Fagan and Poland,[25] which included only house staff and medical students, groups that were expected to be at highest risk of TB exposure. The NIOSH study included a broad spectrum of workers in selected areas of the hospital. Further, the NIOSH study documents a high infection rate among clerical workers, who have patient contact but considerably less than nurses and physicians.

In summary, the NIOSH study at Jackson Memorial Hospital establishes that, for urban hospitals with large numbers of patients with tuberculosis and inadequate controls, the number or workers at risk of acquiring TB infection is large and that the risk of such infection is significant.

CONCLUSION

Recent studies of tuberculosis among occupational groups amply demonstrate that the risk of such infection for health care workers is significant. Documented hospital outbreaks of tuberculosis, including the multidrug-resistant type, have been accompanied by PPD conversion rates of 30–50% among workers attending patients in these outbreaks. Recent surveillance studies show that some groups of health care workers who care for patients with tuberculosis under routine conditions are experiencing annual PPD conversion rates of 5–10%. These rates are clearly higher than the 1–3% annual PPD conversion rates seen in surveillance studies in the 1970s (*see* Table 2).

Acquisition of *M. tuberculosis* is traditionally believed to require *prolonged and intimate contact* with a patient with active pulmonary tuberculosis. Recent occupational studies suggest that this dictum is an oversimplification. Under conditions of intensive exposure to airborne Mtb, such as occurred in the studies of Haley, Hutton, and Catanzaro,[10,28,29] a few hours of contact with a single case of tuberculosis was sufficient for 40–80% of exposed workers to become infected. Nor does it appear that intimate contact with patients with tuberculosis is required for spread of infection. The studies by Ehrenkranz, Hutton and Boudreau[24,29,33–35] amply demonstrate that workers and others with nonclinical contact with tuberculosis patients—less than that which physicians and nurses have with such patients—have significant PPD conversion rates of up to 15–25% in selected studies.

Although the overall incidence of tuberculosis in the United States in the 1970s was higher than it was in the late 1980s and early 1990s,[13] PPD conversion rates in recent surveillance studies and outbreak investigations appear to be higher than the rates in comparable studies in the 1970s. The few exceptions include reports by Catanzaro[10] and Ehrenkranz and Kicklighter.[24] If this phenomenon is true, there are several possible explanations. First, this could be a reporting artifact, or publication bias, in that occupational outbreaks in earlier decades may have been considered less newsworthy than in the past 10 years. Alternatively, the decreased prevalence of tuberculosis infection in the general population, which has accompanied the decline in incidence and mortality of tuberculosis in recent decades, may have resulted in the first generation of workers in whom infection with tuberculosis is the exception rather than the rule. This increased pool of susceptible people would be vulnerable to tuberculosis infection in work settings with inadequate environmental controls and infection control procedures. A third possible explanation is that the distribution of cases of tuberculosis may have changed in the past 2 decades. An increased concentration of patients with active tuberculosis in selected cities or in selected hospitals may increase the intensity of exposure for workers in those settings even if the overall incidence of tuberculosis is unchanged. The result would be outbreaks of infection in selected geographic pockets. Only additional investigations in locations other than those studied to date would provide this information.

While the aforementioned studies elucidate some of the dynamics of occupational risk of tuberculosis, they do not address how widespread the problem of occupational acquisition is. There is currently no national surveillance system for tracking health care workers who become infected with tuberculosis on the job. Occupation has historically not been included on the TB reporting forms. However, even if such forms included occupation, only cases of active tuberculosis are reported, thereby missing the majority of health care workers who become infected with tuberculosis but do not develop active disease in the short term. OSHA's national enforcement guidelines on tuberculosis require that employers report employees who have or develop a positive PPD skin test on the OSHA 200 log (reporting form for occupational injuries and illness). However, these logs are not routinely submitted to OSHA and cannot be readily used as a database for identifying cases and rates of occupational tuberculosis. In addition, the accuracy and completeness of data from such logs would require careful evaluation.

The proposed risk assessment provisions of CDC's 1993 draft guidelines,[16] if included in the final guidelines, would provide an excellent basis for enhancing information about the risk of tuberculosis among health care workers. These guidelines recommend that employers carefully track and compare PPD conversion rates among groups of employees across time and place within the health care facility. While the principal function of this epidemiologic task would be to identify problem spots within the facility, the information yielded would also potentially provide a broad picture of the magnitude and risk factors associated with occupational acquisition of tuberculosis across a wide spectrum of health care settings. The relative effectiveness of the different measures to control the spread of tuberculosis—administrative, environmental, and respiratory protection—also could be evaluated. Our understanding of the occupational health aspects of the resurgence of tuberculosis and its control would thereby be greatly enhanced.

The application of the proposed CDC risk assessment guidelines to health care and related settings other than inpatient hospitals also would significantly increase current knowledge about the risk of tuberculosis for workers in those settings. While not the focus of this chapter, the number of studies of exposure to tuberculosis among workers in prisons, homeless shelters, social service agencies, and drug treatment programs is very limited. The potential size of the population of workers at risk, the heterogeneity of facilities where such workers are employed, and the difficulty in engaging in early identification and treatment of tuberculosis in clients in these settings suggest that separate epidemiologic studies of tuberculosis infection in these settings should be a priority in future research.

Occupational health concerns have not yet received prominent attention during the recent upswing of tuberculosis in the United States. Limited public health resources have understandably been concentrated on controlling tuberculosis among the people most affected, including the HIV-infected, the immigrants, the poor, the homeless, the imprisoned, and the elderly. Some conclude that the resolution of tuberculosis as an occupational health problem will naturally flow from successful public health and clinical efforts to identify early and treat appropriately people with tuberculosis. This view contains some truth but ignores the special opportunities and responsibilities that arise in the workplace. The enhanced application of epidemiologic methods to the specific study of occupational tuberculosis will provide a clearer picture of the nature of the problem and will allow rational evaluation of the success of efforts and resources dedicated to controlling the hazard of airborne *M. tuberculosis* in the workplace.

REFERENCES

1. Aitken WL, Anderson KM, Albert RK: Is the tuberculosis screening program of hospital employees still required? Am Rev Respir Dis 136:805–807, 1987.
2. Ashley MJ, Wigle WD: The epidemiology of active tuberculosis in hospital employees in Ontario, 1966–1969. Am Rev Respir Dis 104:851–860, 1971.
3. Atuk NO, Hunt EH: Serial tuberculin testing and isoniazid therapy in general hospital employees. JAMA 218:1795–1798, 1971.
4. Barrett-Connor E: The epidemiology of tuberculosis in physicians. JAMA 241:33–38, 1979.
5. Beck-Sague C, Dooley SW, Hutton MD, et al: Hospital outbreak of multidrug-resistant Mycobacterium tuberculosis infection: Factors in transmission to staff and HIV-infected patients. JAMA 268:1280–1286, 1992.
6. Berman J, Levin ML, Orr ST, Desi L: Tuberculosis risk for hospital employees: Analysis of a five-year tuberculin skin testing program. Am J Public Health 71:1217–1222, 1981.
7. Bryan CS, McVicker S: Tuberculosis in the community hospital: Lessons from a single year. J S C Med Assoc 73:267–271, 1977.
8. Calder RA, Duclos P, Wilder MH, et al: Mycobacterium tuberculosis transmission in a health clinic. Bull Int Union Tuberc Lung Dis 66:103–106, 1991.
9. Capewell S, Leaker AR, Leitch AG: Pulmonary tuberculosis in health service staff—is it still a problem? Tubercle 69:113–118, 1988.
10. Catanzaro A: Nosocomial tuberculosis. Am Rev Respir Dis 125:559–562, 1982.
11. Centers for Disease Control: Mycobacterium tuberculosis transmission in a health clinic—Florida, 1988. MMWR 38:256–264, 1989.
12. Centers for Disease Control: Guidelines for preventing the transmission of tuberculosis in health-care settings, with special focus on HIV-related issues. MMWR 39(RR-17):1–29, 1990.

13. Centers for Disease Control: Tuberculosis morbidity in the United States: Final data, 1990. MMWR 40(SS-3):23–27, 1991.
14. Centers for Disease Control: Nosocomial transmission of multidrug-resistant tuberculosis among HIV-infected persons—Florida and New York, 1988–1991. MMWR 40:585–591, 1991.
15. Centers for Disease Control: Transmission of multidrug-resistant tuberculosis from an HIV-positive client in a residential substance-abuse treatment facility—Michigan. MMWR 40:129–131, 1991.
16. Centers for Disease Control and Prevention: Draft guidelines for preventing the transmission of tuberculosis in health care facilities, 2nd ed; Notice of comment period. Federal Register 58:52810–52854, October 12, 1993.
17. Chan JC, Tabak JI: Risk of tuberculous infection among house staff in an urban teaching hospital. South Med J 78:1061–1064, 1985.
18. Craven RB, Wenzel RP, Atuk NO: Minimizing tuberculosis risk to hospital personnel and students exposed to unsuspected disease. Ann Intern Med 82:628–632, 1975.
19. Dandoy S, Hansen R: Tuberculosis care in general hospitals: Arizona's experience. Am Rev Respir Dis 112:757–763, 1975.
20. DiPerri G, Cadeo GP, Castelli F, et al: Transmission of HIV-associated tuberculosis to healthcare workers. Infect Control Hosp Epidemiol 14:67–72, 1993.
21. DiPerri G, Danzi MC, DeChecchi G, et al: Nosocomial epidemic of active tuberculosis among HIV-infected patients. Lancet 2:1502–1504, 1989.
22. Dooley SW, Villarino ME, Lawrence M, et al: Nosocomial transmission of tuberculosis in a hospital unit for HIV-infected patients. JAMA 267:2632–2635, 1992.
23. Edlin BR, Tokars JI, Greico MH, et al: An outbreak of multidrug-resistant tuberculosis among hospitalized patients with the acquired immunodeficiency syndrome. N Engl J Med 326:1514–1521, 1992.
24. Ehrenkranz NJ, Kicklighter JL: Tuberculosis outbreak in a general hospital: Evidence for airborne spread of infection. Ann Intern Med 77:377–382, 1972.
25. Fagan MJ, Poland GA: Tuberculin skin testing in medical students: A survey of U.S. Medical school. Ann Intern Med 120:930–931, 1994.
26. Froines J, Wegman D, Dellenbaugh C: An approach to the characterization of silica exposure in U.S. industry. Am J Ind Med 10:345–362, 1986.
27. Gregg DB, Gibson MS: Employee tuberculosis control in a predominantly tuberculosis hospital. J S C Med Assoc 71:160–165, 1975.
28. Haley CE, McDonald RC, Rossi L, et al: Tuberculosis epidemic among hospital personnel. Infect Control Hosp Epidemiol 10:204–210, 1989.
29. Hutton MD, Stead WW, Cauthen GM, et al: Nosocomial transmission of tuberculosis associated with a draining abscess. J Infect Dis 161:286–295, 1990.
30. Kantor HS, Poblette R, Pusateri SL: Nosocomial transmission of tuberculosis from unsuspected disease. Am J Med 84:833–838, 1988.
31. Krarup KC, Scarisbrick DA: Control of tuberculosis in health service workers: The role of the chest radiograph. J Soc Occup Med 39:128–130, 1989.
32. Lanphear BP, Snider DE Jr: Myths of tuberculosis. J Occup Med 33:501–504, 1991.
33. Letter. Boudreau Y: NIOSH correspondence to Joan Otten, Jackson Memorial Hospital. Cincinnati, NIOSH publication HETA 91-187, April 3, 1992.
34. Letter. Boudreau Y: NIOSH correspondence to Joan Otten, Jackson Memorial Hospital. Cincinnati, NIOSH publication HETA 91-187, April 21, 1993.
35. Letter. Boudreau Y: NIOSH correspondence to Joan Otten, Jackson Memorial Hospital. Cincinnati, NIOSH publication HETA 91-187, May 13, 1994.
36. Lundgren R, Norrman E, Asberg I: Tuberculosis infection transmitted at autopsy. Cancer 68:147–150, 1987.
37. Malasky C, Jordan T, Potulski F, Reichman LB: Occupational tuberculous infections among pulmonary physicians in training. Am Rev Respir Dis 142:505–507, 1990.
38. Nardell EA, Keegan J, Cheney SA, Etkind SC: Airborne infection: Theoretical limits of protection achievable by building ventilation. Am Rev Respir Dis 144:302–306, 1991.
39. National Institute for Occupational Safety and Health: Health Hazard Evaluation Ventilation Report, Jackson Memorial Hospital. Cincinnati, NIOSH publication HETA 91-187, November 24, 1992.
40. Occupational Safety and Health Administration: Enforcement policy and procedures for occupational exposure to tuberculosis. October 8, 1993.
41. Parkes WR: Occupational Lung Disorders. 3rd ed. Oxford, England, Butterworth-Heinemann, 1994.

42. Pearson ML, Jereb JA, Frieden TR, et al: Nosocomial transmission of multidrug-resistant Mycobacterium tuberculosis: A risk to patients and health care workers. Ann Intern Med 117:191–196, 1992.
43. Pierce JR Jr, Sims SL, Holman GH: Transmission of tuberculosis to hospital workers by a patient with AIDS. Chest 101:581–582, 1992.
44. Price LE, Rutala WA, Samsa GP: Tuberculosis in hospital personnel. Infect Control 8:97–101, 1987.
45. Raad I, Cusick J, Sherertz RJ, et al: Annual tuberculin skin testing of employees at a university hospital: A cost-benefit analysis. Infect Control Hosp Epidemiol 10:465–469, 1989.
46. Rieder HL, Cauthen GM, Comstock GW, Snider DE Jr: Epidemiology of tuberculosis in the United States. Epidemiol Rev 11:79–98, 1989.
47. Riley RL, Mills CC, O'Grady F, et al: Infectiousness of air from a tuberculosis ward. Ultraviolet irradiation of infected air: Comparative infectiousness of different patients. Am Rev Respir Dis 85:511–525, 1962.
48. Riley RL, Nardell EA: Clearing the air: The theory and application of ultraviolet air disinfection. Am Rev Respir Dis 139:1286–1294, 1989.
49. Ruben FL, Norden CW, Schuster N: Analysis of a community hospital employee tuberculosis screening program 31 months after its inception. Am Rev Respir Dis 115:23–28, 1977.
50. Snider DE Jr: The relationship between tuberculosis and silicosis [editorial]. Am Rev Respir Dis 118:455–460, 1978.
51. Valiante DJ, Rosenman KD: Does silicosis still occur? JAMA 262:3003–3007, 1989.
52. Vogeler DM, Burke JP: Tuberculosis screening for hospital employees: A five-year experience in a large community hospital. Am Rev Respir Dis 117:227–232, 1978.
53. Wells WR: Airborne Contagion and Air Hygiene. Cambridge, MA, Harvard University Press, 1955.

DEBORAH NAGIN, MPH
NICHOLAS PAVELCHAK
MATTHEW LONDON, MS
RONALD P. DEPERSIS
JAMES MELIUS, MD, DRPH

CONTROL OF TUBERCULOSIS IN THE WORKPLACE: ENGINEERING CONTROLS

From the Division of Occupational Health and Environmental Epidemiology
New York State Department of Health
New York, New York

Reprint requests to:
Deborah Nagin, MPH
New York State Department of Health
Division of Occupational Health and Environmental Epidemiology
5 Penn Plaza
New York, NY 10001

The reemergence of tuberculosis as a major public health problem in the United States has resulted in a concomitant concern about occupational risks to selected groups of workers. In particular, workers serving "high-risk" populations are at increased risk for exposure. Outbreaks, many involving multidrug-resistant strains of tuberculosis, have been reported in numerous health care settings, and investigations have generally revealed poor compliance with basic tuberculosis control measures.[5,11,17] Other traditionally non-health care oriented facilities such as correctional facilities and homeless shelters have also experienced outbreaks of occupational TB transmission.[7-9,14]

This chapter will address available engineering methodologies for controlling the transmission of tuberculosis. Because there is a more substantial body of knowledge and experience about environmental controls in health care settings (particularly hospitals), that will be this chapter's focus. It is our hope, however, that this information will also be useful to individuals designing TB control programs in non-health care settings.

To be effective, these controls must be used in conjunction with other elements of a tuberculosis control program, including early identification, isolation, and treatment; conducting a risk assessment for the facility as a whole and for subgroups/areas within the facility; development of administrative procedures and work practices that limit exposures (and limit the numbers of people exposed); effective staff training; medical surveillance of workers; proper use of respiratory protective equipment; and appropriate follow-up of active cases. Because no single intervention can be completely protective, a comprehensive TB control program must coordinate and integrate each of these control elements.

THE CHALLENGE OF TUBERCULOSIS CONTROL IN HEALTH CARE SETTINGS

Health care is provided in a range of settings, including acute care hospitals, outpatient clinics, extended treatment facilities, and other non-hospital-based institutions. From an environmental standpoint, controlling tuberculosis in health care settings often poses technical and financial challenges. Existing ventilation systems in many facilities are often not designed to meet current tuberculosis control recommendations.

During the 1970s, hospitals and other large institutions sought to reduce operating costs through energy conservation measures.[19] These measures included increasing recirculation of air, sealing of windows and other openings to reduce loss of treated air, and operating the ventilation system in cycles rather than continuously. Additionally, as the incidence of tuberculosis declined in most parts of the United States, the need for environmentally secure rooms meeting acid-fast bacilli (AFB) isolation criteria was reduced. The introduction of antibiotic medications in the 1950s, moreover, had a significant impact on the management and prognosis of patients with tuberculosis. Since antibiotic therapy tended to rapidly reduce the infectiousness of most tuberculosis patients, documented nosocomial transmissions became relatively uncommon.[3] Health care facilities, therefore, had less motivation to maintain stringent isolation practices and to monitor AFB isolation rooms for appropriate operation.

With the resurgence of tuberculosis in recent years and with social factors such as increased homelessness and drug abuse contributing to an increased incidence of multidrug-resistant strains of TB, the ability of antibiotic therapy to quickly render most patients non-infectious has been reduced. As a result, many urban hospitals are now faced with the prospect of upgrading or renovating their facilities in order to control nosocomial transmission of TB. Given the scope of these capital projects, serious financial constraints often exist. However, in order to control TB in health care facilities, engineering solutions can (and must) be found.

These challenges to the implementation of feasible and effective controls are likewise present in non–hospital-based clinical settings such as prison infirmaries and outpatient clinics and in other potentially high-risk worksites such as social service agencies and homeless shelters. Many of these facilities, particularly nonclinical settings, were not designed with infection control as a primary objective. For example, in most facilities that have a ventilation system (many do not), the system has been designed primarily for occupant comfort rather than to control the transmission of disease. In these non–hospital-based settings, facilities are challenged to find relatively inexpensive, yet effective, solutions to their disease control problems.

Tuberculosis is not equally prevalent throughout the population. Health care facilities and other workplaces that serve the public need to assess the extent to which they serve individuals from high-risk groups. Groups known to have a higher incidence of tuberculosis include individuals infected with the human immunodeficiency virus or other immunocompromising disorders such as cancer, diabetes, and kidney disease; drug and alcohol abusers; present and past prison inmates; and the homeless. In addition, people who have recently emigrated from areas where TB is endemic or epidemic, such as Asia, Africa, the Caribbean and Latin America, have a higher incidence of TB.[12]

The magnitude of risk to the worker is determined by many factors, including duration and frequency of contact with infectious individuals, proximity to infectious individuals, degree of infectiousness of the individual(s), susceptibility of the worker, extent of effective engineering controls (ventilation, germicidal [ultraviolet] radiation, high-efficiency particulate air [HEPA] filtration units), and appropriate use of respiratory protection. In general, there is greater concern about situations involving repeated, prolonged, and close contact with infectious people in small rooms with poor ventilation. Patients with unrecognized pulmonary or laryngeal TB who are not on effective antituberculosis therapy pose a particular risk because appropriate precautionary measures may not have been employed; for instance, the patient may not have been placed in proper AFB isolation, or the health care worker did not use respiratory protection.[10] This underscores the importance of training for admitting personnel and other staff in order to raise the index of suspicion for TB and to practice early identification and isolation of patients suspected of having TB.

A well-run tuberculin skin-testing program will help to assess the degree of risk for different sub-populations of employees and will also be useful for evaluating the effectiveness of existing engineering controls.

ELEMENTS OF TRANSMISSION

Mycobacterium tuberculosis organisms (Mtb) are rod-shaped, acid-fast organisms about 1–4 μm long and 0.2–0.5 μm wide.[20] While the bacteria can infect a number of organs in humans, pulmonary and laryngeal disease present the greatest risk of transmission. Respiratory droplets containing Mtb may be formed and released into the air when a person with active TB coughs or, sometimes, speaks or sings. When this occurs, larger droplets will fall to the ground or strike another surface rapidly. Once on a surface, these droplets pose little risk of transmission. Smaller respiratory droplets, however, quickly evaporate in the air to form dried residua known as droplet nuclei. These particles are about 1–5 μm in diameter and can remain airborne for prolonged times.[31] Riley showed that droplet nuclei could travel great distances on prevailing air currents.[25] TB bacteria generated in the tuberculosis ward of a Baltimore hospital traveled through a ventilation system and infected guinea pigs in another area. Recent outbreak investigations in health care facilities have also demonstrated this characteristic.[10] Once inhaled, droplet nuclei are small enough to be inspired deeply and may become established in the alveoli, where infection can be initiated. About 50% of droplet nuclei reach the deep lung; the other half are trapped by the nose and upper respiratory tract.[18]

Laboratory studies have shown that TB infection can occur with the inhalation of a single organism.[25] Clinical experience shows that the higher the concentration of viable bacilli in the sputum of a patient and the longer the exposure to that patient, the greater the risk for infection of the health care worker.[10] Other factors determining a patient's infectiousness include degree of coughing, length of time on appropriate medication, and anatomic location of the infection. Patients with laryngeal or pulmonary TB, for example, are usually more infectious than patients with extrapulmonary TB. Among people with pulmonary TB, those with cavitary disease tend to be more infectious. While the data are limited, individuals with HIV infection do not appear to be more infectious than those without HIV infection. In general, the risk may be higher in areas where care is provided to patients before diagnosis and initiation of isolation precautions. Such areas include clinic waiting areas, emergency rooms, and areas where diagnostic or treatment procedures that stimulate coughing are performed.[10]

Covering the patient's nose and mouth with a handkerchief or surgical mask should reduce transmission by capturing droplets before they evaporate to form droplet nuclei.

Certain areas within a health care facility have been identified as presenting increased risk for exposure to tuberculosis due to one or more of the following conditions: (1) medical care is provided to patients with confirmed TB (e.g, isolation rooms); (2) procedures that can aerosolize body fluids (e.g., diagnostic sputum induction, bronchcoscopy, administration of aerosolized pentamidine, endotracheal intubation, dental work, and autopsies) are performed on individuals who may have TB; or (3) the area serves significant numbers of people who are at increased risk of TB (e.g., emergency departments located in an area with a high prevalence of TB).

ENGINEERING CONTROLS

Properly designed, installed, and maintained engineering controls should reduce or eliminate a hazard *before* personal exposure can occur. These controls should (1) contain the contaminant and prevent it from spreading to other parts of the facility, and/or (2) remove the contaminant from the environment either by exhausting, trapping, or killing it. For TB control, these functions are accomplished primarily through the use of ventilation and secondarily through the use of HEPA filtration and/or UV irradiation.

AFB isolation rooms are a prime example of a space where engineering controls have been designed to control the spread of infection. AFB isolation rooms may be established on inpatient medical floors to care for patients with confirmed TB, or set up in areas such as emergency departments to temporarily isolate patients when TB is suspected.

AFB isolation rooms must meet three basic criteria. First, the room must be at negative air pressure relative to adjacent areas to prevent the spread of aerosolized TB bacteria (directional airflow). Second, the room must have adequate ventilation in order to dilute the concentration of contaminants within the room. The American Society of Heating, Refrigerating, and Air Conditioning Engineers (ASHRAE) recommends a minimum of six air changes per hour (ACH), with at least two ACH being fresh, outdoor air.[4] Finally, air from the isolation room must be directly exhausted outside. In most jurisdictions, the discharge point must be at least 25 feet from any windows or building air intakes.

Ventilation

Directional Airflow

Directional airflow is an important element in controlling occupational transmission of tuberculosis. Air moves naturally from one area to another because of pressure differentials. Air molecules in areas with higher (positive) pressure tend to flow to lower (negative) pressure areas, moving along the path of least resistance.

The use of differential air pressures to limit the spread of a contaminant from one area to another has been proven effective in a variety of work settings. In asbestos removal operations, for example, the enclosed work area is under negative pressure in order to prevent the migration of asbestos fibers to other areas.[15] Noncontaminated air flows into the work area rather than the reverse. The pressure gradient during asbestos abatement operations is achieved by using portable, powered exhaust equipment that uses HEPA filters to remove fibers prior to discharge. Alternatively, hospital operating rooms and burn units are maintained under positive pressure so that potentially contaminated air from hallways and adjacent rooms will not be drawn into these more sterile environments.[4]

For tuberculosis control, isolation rooms and special procedure rooms are maintained at negative pressure relative to adjacent hallways and rooms, causing air from these cleaner, adjacent spaces to flow into the TB-contaminated areas. In essence, the contaminant is contained in a discrete area.

Negative pressure may be created by increasing the amount of air mechanically exhausted from the room relative to the amount supplied. The air pressure in the room is reduced until it is lower than in adjacent areas. In general, health care facilities are creating these pressure differentials through (1) installation of an exhaust system dedicated to the isolation room(s), (2) rebalancing or modifying the operation of the existing HVAC system, (3) increasing the exhaust rate through the bathroom exhaust system, or (4) using modular ventilation units that are vented to the outside or into an anteroom.

Air pressure relationships within a large facility such as a hospital are very complex, sensitive to a variety of influences, and therefore in a near-constant state of flux. Relative negative pressure within an isolation room, therefore, can be easily disrupted. Simple things like opening and closing doors and windows in the isolation room or even in adjacent rooms or hallways may alter pressure relationships. Every time the door is opened to a designated negative pressure room, the pressure differential and linear air velocity through the doorway are reduced (or even reversed). Directional airflow at the door may then be additionally compromised by the movement of people in the hallway or entering and exiting the room. In most instances, this momentary lapse in isolation will not result in serious contamination. However, investigations of nosocomial transmissions have identified disruption of negative pressure as a possible contributing factor.[13]

Although this disruption of desired airflow may occur whenever the room is entered or exited, methods are available to minimize the effect. Sensors that are activated when the door is opened can be used. These units may operate either by the breaking of an electrical connection between the door and the frame or may be designed to detect a reduction in pressure differential between the door and the corridor (e.g., a static pressure gauge). A signal is then automatically sent to the exhaust system to increase fan speed, exhausting air from the room at a faster rate and restoring, at least partially, the desired pressure differential.

A second method to safeguard air pressure differentials in a variety of work settings, including biohazard laboratories, clean rooms, and hazardous materials abatement operations, is the installation of an anteroom. In a hospital, an anteroom is generally a small room located between the patient room and the corridor. One must walk through the anteroom in order to access the patient's room. Thus, the anteroom serves as an airlock or buffer to minimize direct exchange of air from the patient's room to the corridor. This result may best be achieved when the anteroom is at an intermediate pressure relationship: at negative pressure relative to the corridor and positive relative to the patient room. By this method, directional airflow is maintained and contaminants that escape to the anteroom are isolated from the corridor by a negative pressure differential. These contaminants may then be either captured by the anteroom exhaust system or drawn back into the isolation room. Optimally, there should be one anteroom per isolation room (no shared anterooms) to limit intermixing of air within the anteroom and possible cross-infection between patients with different patterns of drug resistance.

The anteroom will preferably be equipped with supply and exhaust ventilation and a mechanism that prevents the doors to the corridor and the patient room from being open simultaneously. A manual override option for this mechanism is necessary to allow transport of patient beds and other medical equipment in and out of the patient room and to allow immediate access during a medical emergency. Compliance with applicable fire codes should be verified before installing such a mechanism.

In order to maintain effective isolation, isolation rooms and anterooms should be completely sealed except for the entrance door and operating ventilation ducts. Additional or adjoining doors should be removed and walled-in or sealed around the entire perimeter. If a suspended ceiling system is present, room walls should extend from the floor to the permanent decking above this ceiling to prevent the migration of air from the room via this route.

Because of its critical importance and its susceptibility to loss or disruption, negative air pressure should be monitored on a frequent and scheduled basis; optimally, monitoring should be performed daily while the room is in use. One way to verify through observation the direction of air movement, and hence provide a qualitative indication of differential pressure, is to use a ventilation smoke tube. The smoke tube is an inexpensive, sensitive device for characterizing air movement. Smoke is generated using an aspirator bulb to pass air through a tube packed with smoke-generating chemicals. To monitor an isolation room, the smoke should be generated around the perimeter of the closed door either from the corridor or within the room. As the smoke is carried by air currents, the direction of the airflow can be visualized. The smoke tube may also be helpful in characterizing airflow patterns and air mixing within the isolation room or other areas.

Negative pressure can also be measured using a static pressure gauge such as a manometer. Manometers are commonly incorporated into ventilation fan systems to indicate the load from the filtration media; as the filters become dirty, the static load on the system increases. A manometer can also be employed within the exhaust duct to monitor operation of the fan unit. A malfunction resulting in loss of negative pressure would trigger an audible or visible alarm in the central maintenance station and/or at the appropriate nursing station.

A static pressure gauge also can be installed to measure the pressure differential between the patient room and the corridor and/or anteroom. Negative pressure can then be monitored directly and quantitatively on a continuous basis. Ideally, these monitors would be connected to an alarm or light that would indicate when negative pressure has been breached. However, these systems may pose significant problems if improperly designed or installed. Given the small pressure differentials involved, these gauges need to be highly sensitive and periodically calibrated. Time-dependent circuitry is available to withhold activation of the alarm until negative pressure is lost for a pre-determined period of time—perhaps 30 seconds. This allows for routine activities that result in fluctuations of relative pressure, such as entering and exiting the isolation room, to proceed without setting off the alarm.

When an isolation room is first established or new monitoring equipment is being used, an industrial hygienist or ventilation specialist should try to simulate day-to-day activities to identify aspects that might disrupt negative pressure such as closing the bathroom door or opening the stairwell door. Once negative pressure is stabilized, it should be verified on a regular and frequent basis and records should be maintained. In some facilities, nursing or infection control staff members integrate routine checks into their duties. For TB isolation rooms that are not frequently used, the room should be tested near the time of use and on a daily basis while in use. Negative pressure should be re-evaluated when major renovations, repairs, or ventilation changes have occurred in the building.

Direct Exhaust

In order to assure that air from AFB isolation rooms does not contaminate other areas of the facility, the air should be directly exhausted to outside the building. To prevent the air from reentering the facility, many jurisdictions require that it be discharged at least 25 feet away from any air intake or opening to the building such as doors and windows. Supplemental treatment of the exhaust air using HEPA filtration or exposure to germicidal (UV) radiation may also be considered (see sections on HEPA and UV).

Dilution Ventilation

The methods of negative pressure and direct exhaust are critical for isolating infectious individuals and thereby protecting the rest of the facility. The methods are necessary for AFB isolation rooms but do not provide protection for staff and visitors who enter the isolation room or otherwise share air with an infectious patient. In addition, these methods are often not practical for other parts of the facility, such as emergency departments and outpatient clinics, where infectious TB patients may be present. For both of these reasons, dilutional ventilation should be used, which will reduce the concentration of contaminant within areas where potentially infectious individuals may be located. This is necessary for isolation rooms as well as congregate areas. Dilutional ventilation involves the introduction of a sufficient volume of uncontaminated air into the area to mix with (dilute) and displace the contaminated air. In instances where positive or negative pressurization is required, supply and exhaust airflows should be adjusted accordingly.

Ventilation rates are frequently expressed in terms of air changes per hour, which equates to the number of times a volume of air equal to the volume of the room is ventilated in one hour. The term may be misleading, however, because uncontaminated supply air is simultaneously mixed with the potentially contaminated air being exhausted. The result of this interaction is that one air change does not remove 100% of the contaminant. Theoretically, approximately 63% of the initial contaminant is removed with one air exchange, although the fraction actually removed depends on the extent of air mixing. Incomplete air mixing will result in less than 63% of the contaminant being exhausted. This poor mixing can result in stagnant air or "dead spaces" in the room and is often attributed to and exacerbated by improper placement of the exhaust and supply openings. Introducing a mixing factor is common practice to account for real-world conditions. The factor can vary from one for perfect mixing to 10 for poor mixing. The mixing factor for a specific area can be determined empirically by a qualified industrial hygienist or ventilation engineer. Each subsequent air change will then remove the same percentage (63%) of the remaining contaminant. Table 1 presents the theoretical reductions in contaminant levels. After six air changes, 99.75% of the original contaminant has been removed from the air. The calculations assume perfect mixing—which is only theoretically attainable—and that no new contaminants are being introduced.[1]

Six air changes in 1 hour is equivalent to an air change rate of 6 ACH. Six air changes in one half hour equates to 12 ACH. The current ASHRAE standard for TB isolation rooms is 6 ACH, with at least 2 ACH being fresh (outdoor) air.[4] This standard is based primarily on comfort and general air quality considerations rather than on infection control.

Choosing an Appropriate Ventilation Rate. Ideally, the choice of the appropriate ventilation rate for a particular area should be guided by an assessment of exposure levels in that particular area and by comparing those levels to acceptable safe limits. For Mtb, however, there is no consensus for an acceptable exposure level, nor is the level of contaminant easily measured. Airborne biosampling techniques presently available require culturing of samples over several weeks, and more productive ambient organisms often flourish in the culture medium, making it difficult to accurately count TB colonies.

In the absence of these quantitative tools to evaluate on-site exposure levels, other practical considerations should be used to assist in decision-making. Overall, ventilation rates should be designed for "worst case" scenarios. For example, in a busy, urban emergency department with a high turnover of patients with potential active TB, the ventilation rate for emergency department isolation rooms must be at least sufficient to purge adequately the area of airborne contaminants prior to reoccupancy.

Using six air changes as an arbitrary target (99.75% clearance), the decision of how quickly to provide this degree of contaminant removal needs to be made.

TABLE 1. Theoretical Reduction of Airborne Particles

Air Changes	[C]/[Co]	% Reduction
1	0.37	63
2	0.14	86
3	0.05	95
4	0.018	98
6	0.0025	99.75
9	0.0001	99.99
10	6.1 × 10-6	>99.99
15	3.0 × 10-7	
20	2.1 × 10-9	
25	1.4 × 10-11	

[Co] = initial concentration of particles
[C] = concentration of particles after air change(s)

Table derived from rate of purging equation: VdC = –Q'Cdt,
V= room volume, C = concentration, Q' = effective ventilation rate, t = time and Q' = Q/k, where Q = actual ventilation rate and k = mixing factor.[1]

Assumptions:
1. Instantaneous and perfect mixing within room (k= 1)
2. No additional particles introduced during air exchange(s)

Assessing the frequency of patient turnover will provide guidance in choosing the appropriate ventilation rate for the area. The higher the ventilation rate, the more quickly the room can be safely occupied. Emergency department workers who must enter isolation rooms to care for patients also benefit from these higher rates of dilution ventilation. A table that indicates purge rates at 90, 99, and 99.9% removal efficiencies is reprinted here from the Centers for Disease Control's *Morbidity and Mortality Weekly Report* (Table 2).[10] These values reflect ideal air mixing conditions. Introduction of a mixing factor would normally increase the purge period 3–10 times, especially for large areas or in rooms where it is difficult to achieve good mixing.

In an inpatient AFB isolation room, ventilation rates should also be designed for "worst case" scenarios, meaning highly infectious and symptomatic individuals. In these instances, rapid turnover of patients is not an issue. Instead, the patient remains in isolation for prolonged periods while the health care worker provides ongoing care. The ventilation system serves to dilute the concentration of droplet nuclei in the air but, theoretically, the room will never be completely purged of contamination until the source—the patient—ceases coughing and is rendered noninfectious through drug therapy. While the research is limited, studies suggest that substantially higher rates of ventilation above 6 ACH provide greater reduction of bacteria in a room.[16,27] Increased ventilation rates also have been used for years in operating rooms and other critical care areas to control nosocomial transmissions.

TABLE 2. Air Changes per Hour and Time Required for Removal Efficiencies of 90%, 99%, or 99.9% for Airborne Contaminants[10]

	Minutes Required for Removal Efficiency of		
Air Changes per Hour	90%	99%	99.9%
1	138	276	414
2	69	138	207
3	46	92	138
4	35	69	104
5	28	55	83
6	23	46	69
7	20	39	59
8	17	35	52
9	15	31	46
10	14	28	41
11	13	25	38
12	12	23	35
13	11	21	32
14	10	20	30
15	9	18	28
16	9	17	26
17	8	16	24
18	8	15	23
19	7	15	22
20	7	14	21
25	6	11	17
30	5	9	14
35	4	8	12
40	3	7	10
45	3	6	9
50	3	6	8

Common sense considerations lead to similar conclusions. Using the theoretical removal efficiencies described above as a guide, six air changes would result in 99.75% clearance of the air. As noted, these calculations assume that there is ideal mixing and that no new contaminant is being introduced. In a real-life setting, such as an isolation room, these efficiencies are not expected to be attained. However, even assuming these "best case" or ideal conditions, common sense tells us that approaching 100% clearance of airborne contaminants every hour is too slow. More frequent rapid clearance is required in order to prevent build up of infectious droplets in the air, reduce concentrations, and thereby effectively protect health care workers and visitors who must enter the patient care area on a regular basis. This is particularly important in these "worst case" situations with highly infectious and symptomatic patients.

In isolation rooms, emergency departments, and inpatient wards, workers may be directly exposed to infectious aerosols while in close proximity to a coughing patient. In these instances, dilution ventilation will not provide immediate protection to the workers since it is not a form of local exhaust ventilation, which captures the contaminant at the source of generation before it can be breathed in by another person. As a consequence, additional control measures, most notably a respirator and instructing the patient to cover coughs with a tissue, are necessary.

Supplements to Ventilation

The two primary supplemental environmental control methodologies for TB are air filtration (specifically, HEPA filters) and ultraviolet germicidal irradiation (UV). HEPA and UV are considered interim or supplemental controls to be used in combination with other ventilation measures. As is the case for many TB control measures, there are few published studies documenting the effectiveness of HEPA and UV in preventing tuberculosis transmission, particularly in field rather than laboratory settings. In addition, there are uncertainties about proper deployment, and, most importantly, the effectiveness of these methods is dependent upon the existence of good ventilation. Appropriate dynamic air patterns and a sufficient degree of air mixing are prerequisite to the efficacy of these methods. Air must be moved across the HEPA filter or UV lamp in sufficient quantities to effectively decontaminate the whole space. In the absence of mechanical ventilation, moreover, these methods cannot provide outdoor air that is necessary to maintain acceptable indoor air quality. However, while HEPA and UV should not serve as a primary engineering control measure, they nevertheless play a vital role in TB control.

There are a number of situations for which these methodologies should be considered, including the following:

(1) as an interim measure pending the completion of a large capital improvement project to install or upgrade a ventilation system;

(2) in areas that pose a highly variable risk of TB transmission—rooms that only infrequently have a patient suspected of having TB or rooms housing highly infectious or severely immunocompromised patients; and

(3) as an enhancement to substandard ventilation capacity. In this instance, assuming that both negative pressure and adequate fresh air standards are maintained, HEPA filtration may be particularly appropriate, serving as a substitute for a portion of the exhaust ventilation to achieve a higher equivalency of ventilation in an isolation room.

HEPA FILTRATION

Mechanical filtration has long been employed in a number of occupational settings to control contaminants such as particulate dusts, aerosols, and microorganisms. Filter media vary greatly in capturing efficiency. Given the effective diameter of tubercle bacilli (0.5–3 μm) and droplet nuclei (1–5 μm), the most appropriate filter type is a HEPA filter. HEPA filters remove at least 99.97% of particles 0.3 μm in diameter. Particles with an aerodynamic diameter of 0.3 μm are the most difficult to remove by filtration, and HEPA filters have 99.97% or greater removal efficiency for particles in the size range of droplet nuclei. While no studies have evaluated the effectiveness of HEPA filters in removing TB droplet nuclei from the air, HEPA filters have been shown to be effective in controlling transmissions of *Aspergillus* in the health care setting.[30] These spores (1.5–6 μm) are in the same size range as TB droplet nuclei. In addition, HEPA filters have been used successfully for years in laboratory biosafety cabinets for TB control. While there is general confidence and consensus about the ability of HEPA filters to capture tubercle bacilli, the lack of definitive data underscores their supplemental, yet vital role in TB control. While some manufacturers may market their filters as "HEPA-like" or "high efficiency," it is important to verify that a filter has been tested to meet HEPA criteria (at least 99.97% removal efficiency at 0.3 μm particle size).

The three major applications for HEPA filters in the control of tuberculosis are in (1) ventilation ducts, filtering air before it leaves the building or is recirculated back into the room; (2) modular air filtration units, enhancing existing room ventilation capacity; and (3) portable booths and canopy units, used for special procedures or for temporary isolation.

In-Duct HEPA Filters. This application employs HEPA filtration to solve two different tuberculosis control problems. First, most jurisdictions require that AFB isolation room air not only be exhausted directly to the outside, rather than recirculated, but that it be exhausted at least 25 feet from windows, vents, people, or animals. Where it is prohibitively expensive or infeasible to comply with the "25-foot rule," some facilities are HEPA-filtering the air before directly exhausting it outside. In-duct HEPA filters are also used in emergency departments, clinics, and other congregate settings to filter potentially contaminated air before it is recirculated back into the general ventilation system. Fans used in conjunction with in-duct HEPA filters must be sized to handle the static pressure resulting from the increased resistance provided by a high-efficiency filter.

Proper installation, maintenance, and testing of HEPA filters is critical. There should be adequate space for maintenance personnel to gain access to the filters. In addition, because a potentially serious problem would result from leakage between the filter bed and housing, care should be taken during installation to properly fit and seal the filter to the frame. A quantitative assessment of leakage and filter performance using a dioctyl phthalate (DOP) penetration test should be performed upon installation, at a minimum of six-month intervals and whenever the filter is changed. A manometer or differential pressure gauge should be installed across the filter to monitor static pressure loss as an indicator of filter loading. This will assist in determining when to replace the filter. Installation of a prefilter can prolong the life of the HEPA filter by removing larger particles. The general rule of thumb is that the in-duct HEPA filter should be changed if, with a clean prefilter, the static pressure has increased 2.5 times the initial static pressure reading. Since ventilation systems vary, the design engineers should be consulted regarding criteria for replacement of the prefilter and HEPA filter. A loaded filter can result in a reduced ventilation rate and may also increase the potential for air to bypass the filter. Personnel who change the filters should receive appropriate training and, while there are minimal data regarding the potential hazards of handling the used filters, gloves and a properly fitted respirator should be worn for personal protection. Some facilities have chosen to dispose of these filters as biohazardous waste.

Modular Air Filtration Units. A variety of modular air filtration units are being marketed to help control the transmission of tuberculosis. Modular air filtration units are generally being employed in areas where (1) the existing ventilation capacity is inadequate to meet minimum standards, e.g., emergency department or other congregate settings; or (2) as a supplement to baseline ventilation requirements, providing an extra measure of protection for high-risk patients (e.g., AFB isolation or special procedure rooms). These modular units may be free-standing, wall-mounted, or ducted.

Recirculating air filtration units pull air through a HEPA filter and re-circulate "cleansed" air back into the room. They do not provide negative pressure. Most units are self-contained, modular systems that can be wheeled or carried throughout the facility. The portable nature of these units represents both a strength and weakness. Their portability allows them to be moved within an area if its use or configuration changes, and it allows them to be deployed elsewhere in the facility, if necessary. They can be used in emergency rooms, waiting areas, and clinics to supplement the existing ventilation systems. However, their portability means that they can be inappropriately moved by staff or clients after having been properly placed, and they may be more vulnerable to vandalism or tampering.

Placement of Portable and Wall-Mounted HEPA Units. Proper placement of the unit maximizes the amount of contaminated room air circulating through the HEPA filter. HEPA units should generally not be placed near the air supply, in a corner, near a door, or behind furniture. If possible, the unit should draw air from the patient and away from the health care worker. For example, if most clinical procedures can be performed from the left side of the bed, the unit could be placed near the head of the right side of the bed. Besides optimal ventilation performance, considerations such as excessive noise and drafts should be considered.

Health care workers and patients should be instructed not to place objects such as books, planters, medical devices, and cups on the units. These objects can impede airflow through the unit and may also damage the unit.

Some HEPA units may be mounted on a wall. While this reduces the chance of the unit being tampered with or inadvertently moved, it may also reduce the percentage of contaminated room air drawn through the unit.

Monitoring/Maintenance of HEPA Filters. Monitoring of all HEPA filters should be included in the preventive maintenance program for the facility's existing HVAC system. The preventive maintenance program should include monitoring the static pressure readings across the HEPA filters and inspection of the filters and their seals.

When the unit is installed, it is important to record the initial static pressure at the designated fan speed. This reading can also be taped to the unit for easy reference. Most units have a static pressure gauge to indicate the degree of filter loading. As with in-duct HEPA filters, the system's manufacturer should provide criteria for replacement of the filter(s). If a filter has become excessively loaded, it may cause decreased airflow through the unit and/or increased potential for leakage around the HEPA filter.

Staff who perform the monitoring and maintenance should have a working knowledge of ventilation principles and have experience using ventilation assessment equipment like velometers, anemometers, and manometers. In addition, they should understand how the filters/HVAC system fit into the facility's infection control program.

Use of Air Filtration Units to Obtain Negative Pressure. When a facility has an inadequate number of AFB isolation rooms, two types of products can provide an interim solution: ducted modular units and canopy units.

Ducted Modular Units. Ducted modular units employ a powered exhaust equipped with a HEPA filter. Some units also offer a UV option. Air passes through the filter (and UV field) and is then exhausted through a duct. The duct may exhaust outside or into an anteroom. Some units are equipped with a sensor that detects the door opening, causing a temporary loss of negative pressure in the room. The unit then compensates for this loss by increasing the ventilation rate.

There are a variety of concerns with these units, particularly when they are ducted into an anteroom that is at neutral or positive pressure relative to the corridor or other patient rooms. If there is a failure with the HEPA filtration (leakage around the casing, damaged filter), contaminated air will pass into the anteroom and be readily distributed to the corridor or other rooms. As with all portable HEPA units, their effectiveness depends upon existing room ventilation, particularly good air mixing. Additionally, the units do not provide any fresh air and therefore do not maintain acceptable general air quality.

Canopy Units. Canopy units are essentially an "isolation room within a room." A vinyl tent enclosure is mounted over the patient's bed or over a wheelchair. The tent is under negative pressure and provides at least six ACH (usually much more). Air is passed through a HEPA filter; some units also have a charcoal filter available to adsorb fugitive chemotherapeutic agents. Canopy units are most suitable for bedridden patients, although some facilities are using them in emergency rooms to expand isolation room capacity. They also can be used as a short-term isolation room while permanent rooms are being renovated/constructed. Their use for ambulatory patients is problematic, however, because the canopies are much smaller than a room. Additionally, these units may be suitable for certain special procedures like sputum induction and administration of aerosolized pentamidine, assuming sufficient time is provided between patients to allow for adequate air clearance.

ULTRAVIOLET GERMICIDAL IRRADIATION

Ultraviolet germicidal radiation has been shown to have a lethal effect on a variety of microorganisms, including mycobacterium. Studies have demonstrated the microbial effectiveness of UV radiation in laboratory, clinical, and social settings. The use of UV radiation in the operating theater, for example, has been reported to reduce the incidence of postoperative infections. Wells reported a reduction in the transmission of measles in a public school from the installation of germicidal lamps in hallways and classrooms.[32] Additional studies have suggested ultraviolet radiation to be an effective control measure for TB transmission. A study performed in the late 1950s observed that no guinea pigs became infected by the air exhausted from a tuberculosis ward in a Baltimore hospital when UV radiation was used in the exhaust duct; however, tuberculosis was diagnosed in guinea pigs breathing nonradiated air from the same ward.[25] Although UV radiation has been used as an infection control measure for several decades, the resurgence of TB in the U.S. has sparked a renewed interest and scrutiny into the experimental and experiential indications of its efficacy. One recent study, for example, suggested that some earlier studies may have little predictive value for the level of UV effectiveness that can be expected under a variety of work settings and indoor environmental conditions.[21] This may be related to the factors that determine the microbicidal activity of UV radiation (UV dosage, relative humidity), as well as factors that can affect the output of commercially available UV fixtures (temperature, age of lamp, cleanliness of lamp). These factors, many of which may be difficult to adequately control or predict within a dynamic environment, are discussed within this section and in the appendix to this chapter.

Wavelengths of the electromagnetic spectrum are commonly divided into several regions, including radio, infrared, ultraviolet, x-ray, gamma ray, and cosmic ray. Ultraviolet radiation is characterized as the region of the electromagnetic spectrum between about 15–400 nm. The UV region reported to have microbicidal effects is in the range of 220–300 nm with a maximum at 265 nm.[29] Factors that determine a lethal dose include the wavelength of the germicidal radiation, the density of the radiant flux, the duration of exposure, and the relative susceptibility of the microorganism of interest.[22] About 95% of the transmission from commercially available germicidal lamps is at a wavelength of 253.7 nm.[22]

In addition to the microbicidal effects, UV radiation in the germicidal range may produce undesirable physiological responses in people exposed to direct or reflected rays. This includes a reddening of exposed skin (erythema) and inflammation of the cornea (photokeratitis) and conjunctiva (conjunctivitis).[23] These symptoms are normally not evident until several hours after sufficient exposure occurs and, although painful, are not considered to have long-term effects.[6,26] Similar to the microbicidal dose, the degree of exposure necessary to produce these symptoms is dependent on the wavelength, the density of the radiant flux, the duration of exposure, and the susceptibility of the individual. The American Conference of Governmental Industrial Hygienists (ACGIH) has published Threshold Limit Values (TLV) for occupational exposure to UV radiation. The TLV for the 254 nm wavelength is 0.2 μw/cm^2 for an 8-hour workshift.[2] This recommended limit is directly proportional to the product of the intensity of the radiant field and the duration of exposure. Increasing the field intensity, therefore, decreases the recommended duration of exposure by a proportional amount (Table 3).

Lamp Characteristics. Commercially available germicidal lamps generate UV by passing an electrical discharge through a low-pressure mercury vapor. Electromagnetic radiation is emitted at discrete wavelengths, including 253.7 nm

TABLE 3. Threshold Limit Values for Radiation at 254 nm Wavelength

Irradiance (μW/cm^2)	Daily Exposure (hours)
0.1	16
0.2	8
0.4	4
1.6	1
10.0	0.16

(~95%) as well as wavelengths in the visible band of the spectrum. This visible light is responsible for the characteristic blue glow from these lamps. The germicidal wavelengths are not detectable to the human eye.

The effective output of these lamps may be influenced by several environmental factors as well as inherent properties of their design. Accumulation of dust on the lamp's surface will reduce the radiant intensity. Germicidal UV, moreover, has poor ability to penetrate surfaces, and microorganisms may be shielded by airborne particles. Decreased germicidal effectiveness has also been associated with relative humidities above 65%.[27] According to Sylvania GTE, the germicidal effectiveness of these lamps is optimized in still air and at a temperature of 77° F. Since lamp output tends to depreciate rapidly during the first 100 hours of use, lamps are initially rated at their anticipated 100-hour output level, in still air, at 77° F.[22,29] The expected lifetime of the lamp is generally specified by the manufacturer and will often be as much as 5000 hours of use.

In accordance with the "inverse square law" for electromagnetic radiation, the intensity of UV decreases in proportion to the square of the distance from the source. Doubling the distance from the source, therefore, decreases the intensity of the field by a factor of four. At close distances, however, germicidal tubes do not approximate point sources and Schechmeister suggests that "an inverse relationship [between the intensity and the distance] exists . . . out to about one-half of the effective length of the source."[29]

Applications of UV Lamps. There are three primary applications of germicidal lamps for TB control within facilities: upper-room air radiation, installation of lamps in return air ductwork and/or air plenums, and recirculating room air cleaners.

Upper-Room Air Radiation. Upper-room radiation involves installation of wall- or ceiling-mounted UV fixtures positioned to radiate approximately the upper third of the room. Since room occupants would not be directly exposed to the radiation from properly installed and shielded fixtures, relatively high intensities are used. Factors that may affect exposure include the number and output of lamps, location of lamps, degree of shielding, room reflectance characteristics, and duration of occupancy. To achieve radiation of a significant cross-section of the room volume and to minimize exposure of room occupants to UV, adequate ceiling height must be available. The California Indoor Air Quality Program recommends a minimum ceiling height of 9 feet.[6]

The bacterial effectiveness on airborne pathogens by this method relies significantly on the degree of air mixing between the upper and lower portions of the room. It has been proposed that normal convection currents transport the potentially infectious air present in the lower part of the room to the radiated upper levels at a rate sufficient to provide a substantial reduction in the concentration of viable organisms.[24] Increased vertical mixing has been reported to result in greater disinfection rates. An apparent twofold increase in the rate of disinfection of test organisms was observed by Riley et al. when the ceiling supply air was at least 3° F cooler than the air in the lower part of the room.[28]

Riley and Nardell have reported an equivalent (i.e., to ventilation) room air change rate of 20 air changes per hour (ACH(eq)) for bacille Calmette-Guérin (BCG) using a 30-watt suspended fixture to radiate the upper air in a room with 200 square feet of floor area and 10-foot ceiling height. BCG was described as having similar susceptibility to UV as virulent tubercle bacilli.[26] The authors submit that installation of one 30-watt fixture for every 200 square feet of floor space or every seven occupants may be used as an initial guideline; upper and lower room air mixing, ceiling height, safety, and other factors also must be considered.[26]

In a more recent study of a medical waiting room, Macher et al. state that Riley and Nardell's work has not "shown that this rate of inactivation can be achieved in a ventilated and occupied room in which bacterial aerosols are generated continuously from natural sources." Using a room measuring 90 m^3 (~320 square feet) with a 30-m (~9.8 foot) ceiling, Macher et al. obtained an equivalent air change rate of 1.6 ACH(eq) attributable to four 15-watt wall-mounted germicidal lamps. This rate "was in addition to the 1 to 2.5 ACH that open windows provided and the 8 ACH that the mechanical ventilation system supplied." The authors postulate that the difference between their results and Riley and Nardell's may have been due to a number of factors: The ambient bacteria in their study may have been less susceptible to 254 nm of radiation than the BCG used in Riley and Nardell's experiment; air movement from natural and mechanical ventilation may have reduced exposure times below bactericidal thresholds; and the lower wattage bulbs used may have been less effective despite their increased number.[21]

Additional studies are needed to determine the number, orientation, and output of germicidal lamps to achieve maximum bactericidal effectiveness and to predict the ACH(eq) achievable in specific settings under a variety of conditions such as room shapes and dimensions, rates and characteristics of mechanical and natural ventilation, and number of occupants.

Except for cleaning and changing of the bulbs at indicated intervals, this method is associated with relatively low maintenance. However, monitoring of field intensities and employee exposures requires the purchase of a radiometer with an appropriate 254-nm filter and the availability of a qualified person to take the field measurements and interpret the data.

Ductwork/Plenum UV Fixtures. UV lamps may be installed in return air ductwork and/or plenums to disinfect the air before it is recirculated to that room or another part of the facility. Since these systems are designed to contain the direct and reflected rays within the air handling system, higher intensities may be used.

The volume of air treated in this manner, however, is limited by the capacity of the air handling system. For example, if air is mechanically exhausted from a room at 6 ACH, the upper limit to the rate of disinfection is 6 ACH(eq). Since the lethal dose is dependent on exposure time and field intensity, the velocity at which the contaminated air passes through the irradiated zone must be considered in addition to the number, orientation, and output of the lamps selected.

The use of UV fixtures within ventilation ductwork should not require major renovation of the existing air handling system and/or increased fan horsepower. Except for cleaning and changing of the lamps at indicated frequencies, relatively low maintenance is associated with this method. To prevent significanct employee exposure during maintenance of these units, an automatic power cutoff mechanism should be integral with the maintenance access door. Properly installed germicidal fixtures within return air ductwork and/or plenums reduce the potential for UV exposure of room occupants, as compared to the upper-room air system.

Recirculating Air Cleaners. In a manner similar to duct radiation, the germicidal radiation used by recirculating air cleaners is intended to be contained within the unit. This radiation is usually applied in addition to HEPA filtration or other methods of airborne particle removal. Factors that affect the efficacy of the HEPA filtration units such as air change capability, room air mixing characteristics, and placement of units, are equally applicable to the UV units and the combination UV/filtration units.

The benefit, if any, of supplementing the HEPA filtration with germicidal irradiation in these devices has not been quantified. Assuming 100% disinfection of viable tubercle bacilli captured by the UV or the UV/HEPA units, the maximum theoretical ACH(eq) is determined by the volumetric flow through the irradiation chamber. Although this flow is measurable using a velometer, its value in terms of actual room changes may be less due to room air mixing characteristics.

Except for cleaning and changing the lamps at indicated frequencies, relatively low maintenance is associated with this method. However, since significant employee exposure may occur because of close proximity during servicing of these systems, an automatic power cutoff mechanism should be integral with the maintenance access door.

Maintenance and Monitoring Requirements. A program for periodic monitoring and maintenance of germicidal UV fixtures is critical. The output of germicidal lamps should be monitored on installation and routinely thereafter by qualified personnel using appropriate equipment to verify proper functioning in accordance with the manufacturer's specifications. The lamps should be changed at intervals recommended by the manufacturer or more frequently, if indicated. Records of lamp replacement and of all monitoring should be maintained. Germicidal lamps should be routinely cleaned to prevent accumulation of dust.

In any area where germicidal lamps are present, appropriate monitoring should be performed to quantify personal exposures to UV radiation. Germicidal UV fixtures should be removed, repositioned, or otherwise modified when the potential for overexposure exists or when symptoms of overexposure are present such as skin erythema. Appropriate considerations must be given to the potential for overexposure when installing new fixtures. Records of personal monitoring should be maintained.

Staff members who may be present in areas where germicidal lamps are used should be trained in the potential hazards of exposure to UV radiation, symptoms of overexposure, the operation of the germicidal fixtures, results of applicable personal and area exposure monitoring, proper work practices to minimize the potential for overexposure, and use of appropriate personal protective equipment if applicable. Conspicuous signs should be posted to identify the locations of UV sources. Additional training appropriate to assigned duties should be given to personnel who clean and/or service the germicidal fixtures. These fixtures should be de-energized and locked-out from their power source prior to maintenance or cleaning activities. If the potential for overexposure exists, appropriate personal protective equipment must be worn.

UV Radiation Summary. While some studies indicate that germicidal radiation reduces the number of viable TB droplet nuclei and that this inactivation can be compared to ventilation in terms of equivalent air changes, insufficient information exists to make predictions of the ACH(eq) achievable in specific settings under a variety of conditions. Therefore, germicidal irradiation should not be relied upon to provide a level of protection that is comparable to recommended ventilation parameters.

A lack of consensus exists, for example, on the dose of radiation that is lethal to TB droplet nuclei. Once this dose is established, the minimum field intensities necessary for each of the described applications (upper-air irradiation, ductwork irradiation, air cleaners) may be derived based on the residence time in the irradiated field. This residence time would need to be determined based on the design and air movement characteristics of the specific system. Factors that affect the potential bactericidal activity of germicidal lamps, as described in this chapter and its appendix, must additionally be considered.

While the use of UV as a TB control method is certainly promising, it should not be considered as a primary control method until sufficient information is available to determine the effective dose in all its applications.

High-Risk Medical Procedures

Certain medical procedures pose an increased risk for transmission of tuberculosis, including bronchoscopy, diagnostic sputum induction, administration of aerosolized pentamidine, and endotracheal intubation. In general, such procedures pose an increased risk because (1) they are often performed on individuals with a high risk of tuberculosis, such as AIDS patients, and (2) the procedures themselves promote coughing either by administration of a therapeutic or cough-inducing drug or by insertion of a tube into the patient's throat.

Ventilation Options for High-Risk Procedures

Health care facilities should modify rooms where special procedures are performed to protect staff using the room during and after the procedure. Because of differences among procedures, how they are performed, when they are performed (routine vs. emergency), and where they are performed, all high-risk procedures should be evaluated and control options developed that are tailored to the specific circumstances within an institution. This control plan will require a combination of ventilation controls, respiratory protection, and administrative procedures to minimize the risk of TB transmission.

Current ventilation options available to facilities include the use of local exhaust ventilation and modifying special procedures for rooms to meet at least AFB isolation criteria. When possible, local exhaust ventilation is the preferred engineering control method for high-risk procedures.

Local Exhaust Ventilation. Local exhaust ventilation (LEV) captures the contaminant at the source before it can be dispersed into the environment. The two types of systems on the market designed for high-risk procedures are ventilated enclosures (booths, tents) and exhaust hoods. The ventilated enclosure appears to be used more frequently and is likely to be more protective.

Ventilated Enclosure. If properly installed and maintained, LEV enclosures are ideal for controlling transmission of infectious droplet nuclei. These booths and vinyl tents isolate the patient from the health care worker while the procedure is being performed and until coughing ceases. Air moves by the patient at a high flow rate and is exhausted through a HEPA filter before it is released into the room. After treatment, the patient must stay in the chamber to allow coughing to cease and to help clear the chamber air of aerosols.

To maintain negative pressure conditions throughout the system, the exhaust fan should be located on the discharge side of the HEPA filter to help ensure that contaminated air will not escape to the room and adjacent areas. Because of the high concentration of droplet nuclei often generated during special procedures, it is critical that these booths/tents be functioning as designed. Therefore, regular monitoring and maintenance are essential. A record of these assessments must be kept.

Ventilation Hoods. Ventilation hoods are designed to capture the contaminant at the source where they are generated. Patients receive treatment while sitting in front of and facing into an exhaust hood. Air captured by the system passes through a HEPA filter before it re-enters the environment, or it is ducted directly to the outside. Since these hoods do not fully isolate the patient from the general treatment area, their design is considered inherently less effective than enclosure systems (tents). Hood systems are more susceptible to ambient influences such as adjacent air movement and require proper patient behavior. Adequate capture velocity at the point of contaminant generation is necessary for these systems to be effective.

Maintenance and Certification of LEV Units. While local exhaust ventilation is the optimal control method for high-risk procedures, these systems can be effective only if properly maintained on a regular basis. If filters are damaged or loaded or if units are not well cared for, the equipment may provide a false sense of protection. HEPA filters should be tested and certified at least semiannually. Booths should not be moved unnecessarily. Once moved, their functioning should be assessed and records should be kept of all inspections and testing. Many enclosure units have a static pressure gauge to help monitor directional airflow.

Modifying Special Rooms to Meet AFB Isolation Criteria. In instances where local exhaust options are not feasible or have yet to be developed to meet the requirements of specific procedures, health care facilities should designate certain rooms for special procedures and modify them to meet at least AFB isolation criteria. This includes negative pressure, at least 6 ACH, and proper handling of contaminated exhaust. An example is the construction of bronchoscopy suites.

CONCLUSION

The increased incidence of tuberculosis in the U.S. has heightened concern about possible exposure within certain occupations. Occupational transmissions of tuberculosis have been documented in a number of work settings, and lack of adequate environmental controls has been identified as a contributing factor. Environmental controls are an integral part of a work place-specific tuberculosis control program. These controls are necessary to isolate patients with known or suspected TB from the remainder of the people in the facility. Isolation of infectious individuals is primarily achieved through directional airflow and discharge of potentially contaminated air to the outdoors away from air intakes or areas where people may be exposed. For people who must share space with an infectious individual, protection is provided through dilution ventilation and removal of airborne droplet nuclei, which are primarily accomplished by providing a high rate of air exchange with fresh, uncontaminated air and, secondarily, through HEPA filtration of recirculated air or air disinfection using germicidal radiation. Additional research in the use of engineering control methodologies is needed, particularly with respect to the reduction of risk offered by different levels of dilution ventilation and the methods for predicting the efficacy of the various applications of germicidal radiation. Finally, the use of appropriate respiratory protection is also a part of a facility's TB control program.

APPENDIX: FACTORS AFFECTING DISINFECTION OF MICROORGANISMS BY UV RADIATION

Lamp Output Factors

1. Air Velocity. The output of germicidal lamps varies with the velocity of air flowing past the lamp. In general, the cooling effect of air currents reduces lamp output (the intensity of the field).

2. Temperature of Ambient Air. The output of commercially available germicidal lamps varies with ambient temperature, and manufacturers should provide information on the output of their lamps as a function of temperature. Ideally, the temperature of the air should be maintained to maximize the output efficiency of the selected lamp.

3. Age of Lamp. The output of germicidal lamps depreciates rapidly during the first 100 hours of use, and lamps are generally initially rated at their anticipated 100-hour output level. Although manufacturers provide a rated lifetime for their lamps, the actual output of the lamps should be measured periodically to determine the need for replacement.

4. Cleanliness of lamp. Dust and debris on a lamp's surface can significantly decrease the output intensity.

5. Wattage. The higher the rated power (watts), the greater the anticipated field intensity ($\mu W/cm^2$). Doubling the rated power should give approximately a doubling of the field intensity under similar operating conditions.

6. Reflectance. The field intensity may vary significantly with different reflectance characteristics of surfaces. Reflective indices of common materials are available; however, actual field intensities may be difficult to predict if the number of reflecting surfaces is high and of a variety of materials, the orientation of surfaces is complex, and/or surfaces are of nonuniform reflectance.

7. Inverse square law. The inverse square law states that the intensity of electromagnetic radiation (germicidal UV) generated from a point source in the free field will decrease in proportion to the square of the distance from the source. For example, doubling the distance decreases the field intensity by a factor of four, tripling the distance decreases the intensity by a factor of nine. Since germicidal UV tubes are not point surfaces of light, this relationship is useful for approximations only at large distances from the lamp relative to its length. There is no simple formula for the relationship of field intensity as a function of distance at close distances to the lamp.

Microbial Factors

1. Dose = (field intensity) × (time). The microbicidal effectiveness of germicidal UV is directly dependent on the dose of UV received by the microorganism relative to its susceptibility at the wavelength used. The dose is a product of the field intensity and the time of exposure at that intensity. Since the intensity of the radiant field would not be uniform in location (as a result of the inverse square law, local reflectance), the actual dose received would be the cumulative or time-weighted effect of multiple exposures. Predicting the field intensity necessary to produce a lethal effect, therefore involves understanding:

(i) the lethal dose for the microorganism of interest,

(ii) the field intensity as a function of location, and

(iii) the location of the microorganism in the radiant field as a function of time.

Achieving disinfection, therefore, requires knowledge of (i) and the ability to control, or at least predict, (ii) and (iii). Presently, there is no consensus on the dose of germicidal UV that will consistently kill *Mycobacterium tuberculosis.*

The field intensity, as a function of location, may be determined through direct measurements and mapping of intensity lines. Since these values can be expected to change with time (due to lamp aging, lamp cleanliness, diurnal and seasonal temperature variations), periodic measurements and meticulous maintenance is essential.

Since TB droplet nuclei are carried by air currents, the location of the microorganism in the radiant field as a function of time is determined by the dynamics of air movement in the environment of interest. Controlling or predicting air movement within ductwork may be relatively straightforward; however, air movement within occupied rooms and the factors that affect it are often complex. A simple smoke test may provide a qualitative indication of air movement during a relatively short test period. Using a tracer gas technique can provide a quantitative depiction of air movement characteristics over longer times. This method, however, requires specialized equipment and trained and experienced personnel.

a. Size of field. The germicidal field should be of sufficient size to irradiate all droplet nuclei carried by the air currents. Germicidal lamps used in ductwork should irradiate the entire cross-sectional area and should be placed in a long, straight section of ductwork to maximize the volume of the field.

When wall- or ceiling-mounted units are used in rooms, they should be positioned to maximize the upper-air volume that they irradiate. In general, the lower in height that they are positioned, the larger the overhead "irradiation chamber" created. This principle, however, must be balanced with the need to maintain safe exposure levels to UV for room occupants.

b. Residence time in field/air mixing. Air distribution must be balanced to maintain good air mixing and/or directional airflow to bring the microorganisms into the irradiated field at a sufficient rate, but the microorganisms must be held in the field long enough to obtain a lethal dose.

Germicidal lamps used in ductwork should be placed where the air velocity is slow to obtain sufficient residence time (after the filter bank). This parameter needs to be balanced with the need to maximize the field size as described above.

Room air mixing considerations are important to ensure that a sufficient volume of air is directed to and captured by the exhaust air duct when the duct-irradiation method is used and, similarly, to ensure sufficient vertical mixing of air when wall- or ceiling-mounted fixtures are used. As indicated above, room air mixing dynamics are usually complex, difficult to quantitatively evaluate, and even more difficult to control and/or predict over time.

2. Humidity. Studies indicate that the microbicidal activity of germicidal lamps declines precipitously when relative humidities exceed about 65%.

3. Repair mechanisms. There are three primary mechanisms identified by which bacteria may be repaired following cellular damage from UV radiation. These mechanisms are called excision repair, photoreactivation, and post-replication repair. Bacteria may receive sufficient UV exposure to be damaged, but not rendered inviable. In instances where positive or negative pressurization is required, supply and exhaust airflow should be adjusted accordingly.

REFERENCES

1. American Conference of Governmental Industrial Hygienists: Industrial Ventilation: A Manual of Recommended Practice, Lansing, MI, American Conference of Governmental Industrial Hygienists, 1988.
2. American Conference of Governmental Industrial Hygienists: Threshold limit values and biological exposure indices for 1991–1992. Cincinnati, American Conference of Governmental Industrial Hygienists, 1992.
3. American Hospital Association, Technical panel on infections within hospitals: Tuberculosis Control in Hospitals. Chicago, American Hospital Association, January 1992.

4. American Society of Heating, Refrigerating, and Air Conditioning Engineers: 1991 Applications Handbook. Atlanta, American Society of Heating, Refrigerating, and Air Conditioning Engineers, 1991.
5. Calazaro A: Nosocomial tuberculosis. Am Rev Respir Dis 125:559–562, 1982.
6. California Indoor Air Quality Program: Using ultraviolet radiation and ventilation to control tuberculosis. Berkeley, CA, California Department of Health Services, 1990.
7. Centers for Disease Control: Tuberculosis control among the homeless—Boston. MMWR 34:429–431, 1985.
8. Centers for Disease Control: Tuberculosis control among homeless populations. JAMA 257:286–287, 1987.
9. Centers for Disease Control: Prevention and control of tuberculosis in correctional institutions: Recommendations of the Advisory Committee for Elimination of Tuberculosis. MMWR 38:313–320, 1989.
10. Centers for Disease Control: Guidelines for preventing the transmission of tuberculosis in health care settings with special focus on HIV-related issues. MMWR 39(RR-17):1–28, 1990.
11. Centers for Disease Control: Nosocomial transmission of multidrug-resistant tuberculosis to health care workers and HIV-infected persons in an urban hospital—Florida. MMWR 39:718–722, 1990.
12. Centers for Disease Control: Screening for tuberculosis infection in high-risk populations, and the use of preventive therapy for tuberculosis infection in the United States: Recommendations of the Advisory Committee for Elimination of Tuberculosis. MMWR 39(RR-8): 1990.
13. Centers for Disease Control: Nosocomial transmission of multidrug-resistant tuberculosis among HIV-infected persons—Florida and New York. 1988–91. MMWR 40:585–591, 1991.
14. Centers for Disease Control: Transmission of multidrug-resistant tuberculosis among immunodepressed persons in a correctional system—New York 1991. MMWR 4(28):507–509, 1992.
15. Code of Federal Regulations: 29 CFR 1926.58. Office of the Federal Register, National Archives and Records Administration. U.S. Government Printing Office, Washington, DC.
16. Galson E, Goddard KR: Hospital air conditioning and sepsis control. ASHRAE Journal, July 1968, 33–41.
17. Haley CE, McDonald RC, Rossi L, et al: Tuberculosis epidemic among hospital personnel. Infect Control Hosp Epidemiol 10:204–210, 1989.
18. Hatch TF: Behavior of microscopic particles in the air and in the respiratory system. Aerobiology 17:102–105, 1942.
19. Health Resources and Services Administration: Guidelines for Construction and Equipment of Hospital and Medical Facilities, 1983–84. US Dept of Health and Human Services publication (HRS-M-HF) 84-1.
20. Jolik WK, Smith DT (eds): Zinsser Microbiology. 15th ed. New York, Meredith Corp., 1972.
21. Macher JM, Alevantis LE, Chang Y-L, Liu K-S: Effect of ultraviolet germicidal lamps on airborne microorganisms in an outpatient waiting room. Appl Occup Environ Hyg 7:505–513, 1992.
22. Mpelkas CC: Germicidal and short-wave ultraviolet radiation. Danvers, MA, Sylvania GTE, 1983, GTE Products Corporation engineering bulletin 0–342.
23. National Institute for Occupational Safety and Health: Criteria for a recommended standard: Occupational exposure to ultraviolet radiation. Cincinnati, 1972, US Dept of Health, Education, and Welfare, publication HSM 73-11009.
24. Riley RL: Airborne infection. Am J Med 57:466–475, 1974.
25. Riley RL, Mills CC, Nyka W, et al: Aerial dissemination of pulmonary tuberculosis: A two year study of contagion in a tuberculosis ward. Am J Hyg 70:185–196, 1959.
26. Riley RL, Nardell EA: Clearing the air: The theory and application of ultraviolet air disinfection. Am Rev Respir Dis 139:1286–1294, 1989.
27. Riley RL, O'Grady F: Airborne Infection: Transmission and Control. New York, Macmillan, 1961.
28. Riley RL, Permutt S, Kaufman JE: Arch Environ Health 22:202–207, 23:35–39.
29. Shechmeister IL: Sterilization by ultraviolet radiation. In Block S (ed): Disinfection, Sterilization and Preservation. 4th ed. Philadelphia, Lea & Febiger, 1991.
30. Sheretz RJ, Belani A, Kramer BS, et al: Impact of air filtration on nosocomial Aspergillus infections. Am J Med 83:709–718, 1987.
31. Wells WF: On airborne infection. Study II, Droplets and droplet nuclei. Am J Hyg 20:611, 1934.
32. Wells WF, Wells MW, Wilder TS: The environmental control of epidemic contagion. I. An epidemiologic study of radiant disinfection of air in day schools. Am J Hyg 35:97–121, 1942.

THOMAS K. HODOUS, MD
CHRISTOPHER C. COFFEY, MS

THE ROLE OF RESPIRATORY PROTECTIVE DEVICES IN THE CONTROL OF TUBERCULOSIS

From the Division of Safety Research
National Institute for Occupational Safety and Health
Morgantown, West Virginia

Reprint requests to:
Thomas K. Hodous, MD
Division of Safety Research
National Institute for Occupational Safety and Health
Morgantown, WV 26505

This article is not a statement of current or proposed NIOSH policy but presents a review of various evolving perspectives and recommendations regarding personal respiratory protection against tuberculosis.

The role and selection of respiratory protective devices* in the control of tuberculosis has recently been the subject of much debate. The traditional use of surgical masks in this setting has been seriously challenged by a number of organizations, including the Centers for Disease Control and Prevention (CDC),[12] the National Institute for Occupational Safety and Health (NIOSH),[60] and, perhaps most importantly because of its enforcement authority, the Occupational Safety and Health Administration (OSHA).[62-63] This debate is in part due to the lack of adequate data regarding a number of issues, including the precise characterization of TB aerosols and their infectivity; the effectiveness of the various respiratory protective devices against these bioaerosols; and the effectiveness of engineering controls as discussed in the preceding chapter. In addition, the involvement of workers in recent TB epidemics in health care and correctional facilities has substantially increased the concern and involvement of the federal occupational safety and health community with the health care industry. Given the different orientations and disease control paradigms of the various occupational

* The term *respiratory protective device* will be used in this chapter to include any covering of the nose and mouth, including both surgical masks and *respirators*. *Respirator* will be reserved for devices designed, certified, and commonly used in various industrial settings to protect the wearer from respiratory hazards.

and health care communities, it is not surprising that alternate risk-management approaches have evolved.

It is useful for the occupational safety and health professional to understand the various arguments in this ongoing discussion. Although future policy changes may occur, federal OSHA regulations of October 1993 requiring high-efficiency filters for personal respiratory protection against TB places substantial new burdens on health care providers.[63] This chapter will describe both surgical masks and respirators and discuss the major issues in their application to TB control. It will then review several recommendations and their rationales and conclude with a view of future directions in this area. Because most readers will be relatively unfamiliar with the practice of respiratory protection in general industry, this area will be emphasized.

RESPIRATORY PROTECTIVE DEVICES

Surgical Masks

As their name suggests, surgical masks (Fig. 1) were originally developed to prevent the wearer's spoken or coughed secretions from contaminating an operative field.[9] However, these devices also have been used for decades to protect the wearer from exposure to various infectious agents, including TB.

Standard surgical masks are considered a Class II device by the federal Food and Drug Administration (FDA), which requires premarket sales approval.[19] To obtain an approval, the manufacturer must demonstrate to the satisfaction of the FDA that the new device is substantially equivalent to similar masks currently on the market. There is no specific requirement to prove that the existing masks are efficacious, and there is no standard test or set of data required to support the assertion of equivalence. Approval requires that good manufacturing practices are followed and allows for periodic inspection by the FDA of the manufacturing process and program. The FDA itself does not conduct or sponsor any testing of surgical masks.

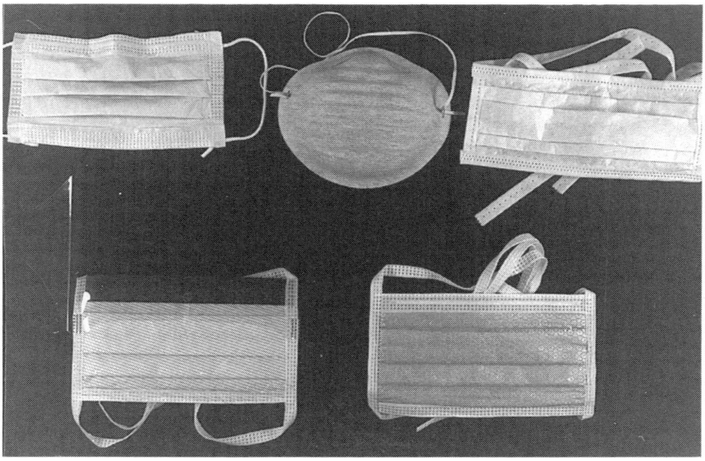

FIGURE 1. Surgical masks. The two lower masks are designed to protect the wearer from airborne occupational hazards such as laser plumes.

Concerns regarding the use of surgical masks for protection against TB are numerous. Traditionally masks were not designed to protect the wearer. Although much research and testing, including biological testing, have been performed by manufacturers and other groups,[33,80] surgical masks legally do not need to be tested for their efficiency.[28] They generally do not permit reliable fit tests or fit checks (see below). Finally, studies have shown variable and sometimes large leakage both around and through the devices.[14,17,35,64,76,81] These findings led the CDC in 1990 to recommend the use of respirators as superior protective devices against TB aerosols.[12]

In the past decade, manufacturers have developed surgical masks intended to protect the wearer from respiratory hazards such as laser plumes. These so-called "protective" surgical masks[4] may be substantially better than standard surgical masks, particularly with regard to filter efficiency and perhaps to face seal. However, there is no standard by which to assess these features, and the deficiencies noted with standard masks remain.

Respirators

The field of personal respiratory protection is complex, sometimes controversial, and evolving. The following sections will attempt to describe the major industrial hygiene tenets in this area. Interested readers are referred to recent reviews[30,44] and more complete sources.[6,26,37,58,59,65]

Both NIOSH and OSHA were created by the Occupational Safety and Health Act of 1970, and both agencies have responsibilities in the area of respirators. The primary responsibility of OSHA is to regulate the use of respirators. The general respirator standard of OSHA[24] requires the use of NIOSH-approved or NIOSH-certified respirators as well as the implementation of a full respirator program. The OSHA standards carry the force of law.

The certification program for respirators is the responsibility of NIOSH, as established under the authorization of the Coal Mine Health and Safety Act of 1969 and the Federal Mine Safety and Health Act of 1977. All respirator certifications currently are jointly issued by NIOSH and the Mine Safety and Health Administration (MSHA). The certification program is designed to help increase worker protection from airborne hazards by ensuring that respirators meet certain minimum performance requirements. These minimum requirements are contained in Title 30, Code of Federal Regulations, Part 11 (30 CFR 11).[25]

The certification program consists of the following components:[25,59]

- Laboratory evaluation of the respirator
- Evaluation of the manufacturer's quality control (QC) plan
- Off-the-shelf audit testing of certified respirators
- In-plant manufacturing QC audits
- Investigation of problems with certified respirators

The requirements in 30 CFR 11 are for issuing certifications to respirators used in mining and general industry. There are no provisions for specifically certifying respirators for use against biological agents such as *Mycobacterium tuberculosis*. However, it is assumed that the standard industrial hygiene practices in selecting an appropriate respirator would apply to all types of aerosols. (A more detailed discussion of this issue is presented later in this chapter.) The approval label (Fig. 2) that appears on each certified respirator lists the limitations and cautions that the wearer should take into consideration when using that respirator.

PERMISSIBLE

POWERED AIR PURIFYING RESPIRATOR FOR DUSTS, FUMES, MISTS, AND RADIONUCLIDES

MINE SAFETY AND HEALTH ADMINISTRATION
NATIONAL INSTITUTE FOR OCCUPATIONAL SAFETY AND HEALTH

APPROVAL NO. TC-21C-495

ISSUED TO
MINE SAFETY APPLIANCES COMPANY
Pittsburgh, Pennsylvania, U.S.A.

LIMITATIONS

Approved for respiratory protection against dusts, fumes, and mists having a time-weighted average less than 0.05 milligram per cubic meter, asbestos-containing dusts and mists, and radionuclides.

Not for use in atmospheres containing less than 19.5 percent oxygen.

Not for entry into atmospheres immediately dangerous to life or health.

Not evaluated as an ignition source in flammable or explosive atmospheres by MSHA/NIOSH.

If using a 7-753-1, 7-753-2, or 7-753-3 facepiece, the D/PD exhalation valve must remain in the "OUT" position.

When using the 495747 cap, plug assembly in the 495692 filter inlet, approval is maintained for egress only.

CAUTION

Replace filter when the air flow falls below 4 cubic feet per minute.

In making renewals or repairs, parts identical with those furnished by the manufacturer under the pertinent approval shall be maintained.

Follow the manufacturer's instructions for changing filter.

This respirator shall be selected, fitted, used, and maintained in accordance with the Mine Safety and Health Administration, Occupational Safety and Health Administration, and other applicable regulations.

MSHA-NIOSH Approval TC-21C-495
Issued to Mine Safety Appliances Company

The approved respirator consists of the following MSA parts: 7-842-1, 7-842-2, 7-842-3, 7-934-1, 7-934-2, or 7-934-3 facepiece, or 7-203-1, 7-203-2, 7-203-3, 7-753-1, 7-753-2, or 7-753-3 facepiece less 96547 breathing tube adapter; 487884 motor-blower assembly; 7-977-1, 9961, 473902, or 487446 belt; 487803 battery; 487807, or 495692 (TC-21C-495) filter; 492944 pre-filter (accessory); and 492941 cover, or 496342 cover with 496341 plenum (accessory).

FIGURE 2. A NIOSH approval label.

In addition, NIOSH makes recommendations on issues dealing with the use of respirators, such as maintenance, assigned protection factors, selection, and fit testing.[59] Unlike the OSHA regulations, these are recommendations only and are not binding on the user of the respirator.

Another important organization that has standards on respirators is the American National Standards Institute (ANSI).[6] ANSI is a consensus organization, and its standards are also recommendations only unless they are specifically incorporated into OSHA regulations.

Types of Respirators

There are two main classes of respirators, based on how they provide protection to the respiratory system. The first class is air-purifying respirators, which remove contaminants from the ambient air. The second class is atmosphere-supplying respirators, which provide the wearer with a source of air other than the surrounding atmosphere.

The two main respirator classes can be further divided by the type of face piece that is used on the respirator. A half-mask respirator fits over the nose and under the chin. A full face piece covers most of the face—from about the hairline to under the chin—thus providing eye protection (Fig. 3).

Two related additional characteristics are the material of the face piece and whether the respirator is disposable. The face piece of most respirators is made of an elastomeric (rubber-like) material. These respirators typically have replaceable parts, including filters, and are reusable. In contrast, some half-mask air-purifying respirators use the filter material itself as the face piece (as with a surgical mask). These respirators are considered disposable (Fig. 4). However, to complicate matters, some elastomeric half-mask air-purifying respirators are variably disposable. They may have no replaceable parts, with other styles having replaceable filters only. Examples of two disposable elastomeric half-masks, as well as a typical reusable elastomeric half-mask respirator, are shown in Figure 5. To avoid confusion with typical uses of the terms, this chapter will consider "disposable" respirators as only those with nonelastomeric filtering face pieces. Elastomeric face piece respirators are generally considered more sturdy and better fitting than disposable masks and have been shown to be more protective in some studies.[43]

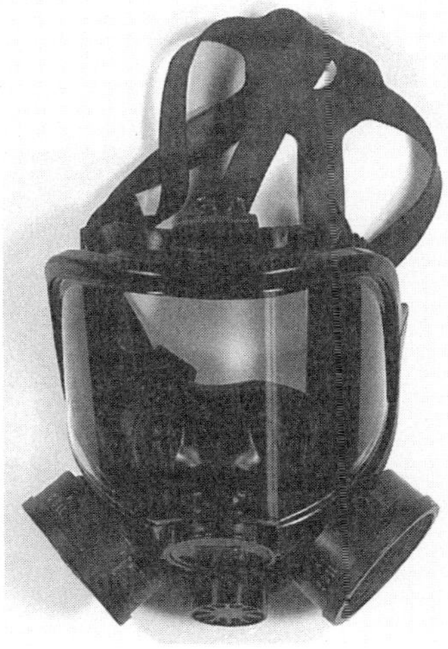

FIGURE 3. Full face piece respirator (all with replaceable filters).

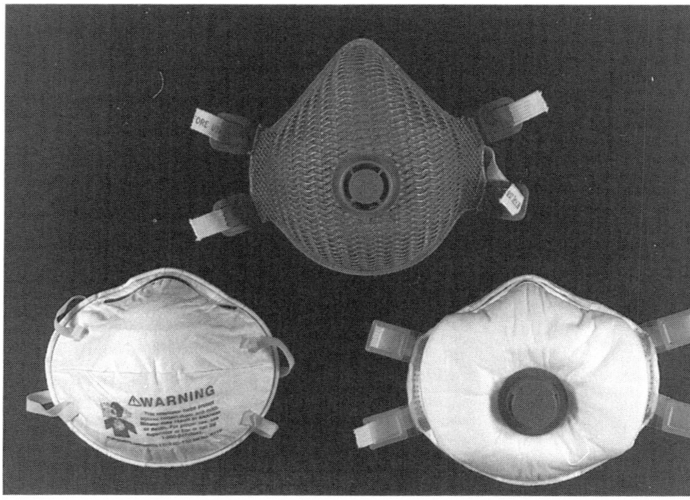

FIGURE 4. Disposable half-mask respirators: dust, fume, and mist (top); dust, mist (bottom left); high-efficiency (bottom right). The DFM and HEPA shown here have exhalation valves, which permit easier exhalation. These are all particulate respirators.

A feature of many but not all respirators is one or more exhaust valves (*see* Figs. 4 and 5). These one-way valves allow the wearer to exhale through the smaller resistance of the valve orifice, reducing the work and discomfort of exhalation.

Air-purifying Respirators

Air-purifying respirators can be further classified by the type of contaminant they can remove. The three main subcategories of air-purifying respirators include the ability to remove either particulates, gas and vapors, or both particulates and gas and vapors. Particulate-removing respirators use a number of different filters that are certified for a variety of dusts, mists, and fumes. Protection from TB aerosols requires a particulate-removing air-purifying respirator. (Gas- and vapor-removing respirators are certified for a variety of gases and vapors but do not provide protection against TB.)

Air-purifying respirators also can be classified by their mode of operation. Nonpowered respirators use the wearer's inhalation cycle to move ambient air through the filters. A powered air-purifying respirator (PAPR) uses a blower to force the ambient air through the filters to the face mask (Fig. 6). Therefore, a positive pressure is produced inside the face piece under most conditions. The flow rate that can be produced by the PAPR (more than 115 liters per minute[25]) exceeds the inhalation flow rates expected in the great majority of workers who need personal respiratory protection against TB droplet nuclei.

Atmosphere-supplying Respirators

Atmosphere-supplying respirators consist of two classes: self-contained breathing apparatus (SCBA) and supplied-air respirators (SAR). The wearer of a SCBA carries the source of respirable air with him/her, often as a compressed air cylinder, as is frequently seen on the backs of firefighters. With a SAR, the source of respirable air is connected to the face piece by up to 300 feet of airline hose.

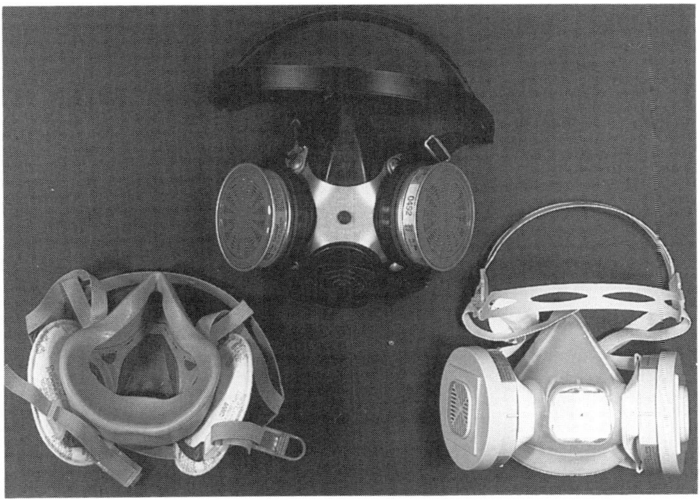

FIGURE 5. Elastomeric half-masks respirators: reusable with replaceable filters (top); disposable except that filters can be replaced (bottom left, shown from face side to show face seal); disposable (bottom right).

A SCBA can be either open-circuit (the wearer's exhaled breath is exhausted to the ambient atmosphere) or closed-circuit (the wearer's exhaled breath is scrubbed of carbon dioxide and rebreathed, with various mechanisms to ensure adequate oxygen). Both types of SCBA, and the SAR, can operate in the demand or pressure-demand mode. In the demand mode, respirable gas is

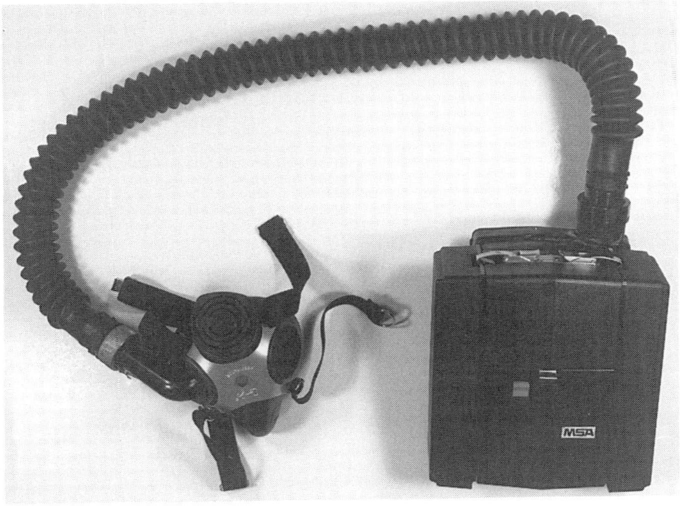

FIGURE 6. Half-mask powered air-purifying respirator with high-efficiency filters (all replaceable). This one has a tight-fitting mask. The air blower and filters form the box-like module that in this case is worn on a waist belt, and the hose carries the purified air to the face piece.

admitted to the face piece only when a negative pressure is created inside the face piece by inhalation. In the pressure-demand mode, the respirable gas is admitted to the face piece when the positive pressure is reduced (but not down to ambient pressure) inside the face piece by inhalation. The latter configuration offers the highest protection of any respirator, since any face seal leakage will tend to be outward. A SAR can also operate in a continuous flow mode in which a constant flow of air is supplied to the wearer regardless of the breathing cycle.

Protection Afforded by Respirators

The level of protection afforded by a particular class of respirators is given by its assigned protection factor (APF). An APF is a measure of the anticipated workplace level of respiratory protection that would be provided by a properly functioning respiratory or a class of respirators to a stated percentage of properly fitted and trained users.[6,34,59] The APF is a special application of the general protection factor (PF) concept. The PF is the ratio of the amount of contaminant to which a person would be exposed without a respirator to the amount of contaminant to which a person is exposed with a respirator. This is determined by comparing the amount of contaminant inside the face piece, C_i, to the amount of contaminant outside of the face piece, C_0. That is:

$$PF = C_o/C_i$$

Since $C_i \leq C_o$, the protection factor is always equal to or greater than unity.

In brief, most current APF values for the various types of respirators are based on (1) extensive research done by Los Alamos Scientific Laboratories under administration of the University of California, in the 1970s[43]; (2) a number of more recently published and presented research studies on APF values;[11,29,46,47,54,55,70,73] and (3) the interpretations of these and other data by expert committees. As might be expected, there are some differences among various national institutions in these values.

The OSHA APF values are listed in Table 1. These values were taken from the most recent OSHA agent-specific standard that listed a particular respirator; the APFs given in other agent-specific standards promulgated earlier than those referenced in Table 1 may be different. OSHA uses the values given in Table 1 for agents not having a specific standard. Both NIOSH[61] and ANSI[6] have recommended APFs, which differ slightly from each other and from those shown in Table 1. The OSHA values have legal authority, although current OSHA regulations[24] still state that proper selection of respirators shall be made according to the guidance of the ANSI Z88.6-1969 document.[5]

Respirator APF values allow the relative protection of different types of respirators to be determined. However, the best quantitative use of APF values occurs when both the ambient level of an airborne hazard and an acknowledged safe level are known. In these cases, a specific type of respirator can be easily chosen to ensure worker protection. For example, if the ambient hazard level is 20 units, and the known safe level is 1 unit, then a respirator with an APF of at least 20 will be needed. Unfortunately, in the case of TB exposure, neither of the two required numbers can be easily measured or are known at the present time. Therefore, respirator APF values are currently of limited use in selecting respirator types for protection from TB.

TABLE 1. Occupational Safety and Health Administration Assigned Protection Factors*

Respirator Type	Respiratory Inlet Covering (Face Piece Type)		
	Half-Mask	Full Face	Hood/Helmet§
Air-purifying			
Disposable	5†	—	—
Non-disposable	10‡	50‡	—
Atmosphere-supplying			
SCBA (demand)	10‡	50‡	—
Airline			
Demand	10‡	50‡	—
Continuous flow	50‡	250‡	25‡
Powered air-purifying	50‡	250‡	25‡
Atmosphere-supplying			
Airline			
Pressure demand	1,000‡	1,000‡	—
SCBA			
Pressure demand	—	1,000‡	—

* See text for explanation of terms. Different protection factors may be found in some older OSHA agent-specific regulations.[20,21]
† From Title 29, Code of Federal Regulations, Part 1910.1043[23]
‡ From Title 29, Code of Federal Regulations, Part 1910.1027[22]
§ OSHA includes loose-fitting face piece respirators in this group.

Respirator Filter and Face Seal Leakage

All air-purifying respirators certified for use against particulates have two ways for the particulate to enter the face piece: face seal leakage and filter penetration. A proper seal between a respirator's sealing surface and a wearer's face is essential for the negative-pressure respirator to provide effective and reliable protection. The seal is less critical but still important for the powered air-purifying respirator. Face seal leakage can be caused by a number of factors, such as incorrect face piece size or shape, incorrect or defective face piece sealing surface, any beard growth on the wearer, slippage of the face piece due to perspiration or oils on the skin, and incorrect donning or maintenance.

To help assure that the seal is adequate, fit testing is required by OSHA to be performed initially and periodically to detect any face seal leakage.[24] Fit tests should help ensure that each wearer has adequate protection and that the selected respirator is properly fitted. Thus, the primary role of fit testing is to ensure that the wearer has selected a respirator size and brand that properly fits his or her face. Fit tests are designed so that the filter penetration of the test substance is negligible.

Standard industrial hygiene recommendations and OSHA regulations[24] require respirator wearers to be capable of effectively and reliably checking their respirator for proper fit before each use. This is to assess point-of-use factors that can create leakage even of a properly selected respirator when the respirator is worn in the work environment.

Currently, NIOSH certifies three types of particulate filters: dust and mist (DM) respirators; dust, fume, and mist (DFM) respirators; and high-efficiency particulate air (HEPA, or high-efficiency) respirators. The DM respirators are not tested for face seal leakage during the certification process. DFM and HEPA respirators are qualitatively fit tested.[25]

Rationales for APF Values

The following discussion explains some of the rationales behind the different APF values noted in Table 1 for various respirators, and it notes factors relating to the proper selection of a respirator for TB protection. Nonpowered respirators have one major limitation that reduces the level of protection they are capable of providing: face seal leakage. During each inhalation by the wearer, a negative pressure (relative to the surrounding air) is created in the face piece. Contaminated air can enter the face piece through leaks, the path of least resistance, avoiding the higher resistance filter material due to this negative pressure.

Accumulated data indicate that half-mask nonpowered respirators have the potential of allowing up to 10–20% leakage around the face seal.[6,27,29,32,43,46] In contrast, data show that the tight-fitting PAPR half-mask respirator, because of the positive pressure inside the face piece under most conditions, has 2% or less face seal leakage.[46] Because of the better probability of a good face seal, tight-fitting full face–piece respirators are also shown to have 2% or less face seal leakage.[43,61] Therefore, the latter two respirators can be safely used in concentrations of a contaminant five times greater than that for a negative-pressure half-mask respirator.

The second source of leakage into a respirator is filter penetration. Current regulations specify testing of DM and DFM filters for penetration using silica dust, lead fume (DFM only), and silica mist.[25] Unfortunately, these tests are associated with several deficiencies, especially in regard to their ability to predict filter penetration of TB droplet nuclei. The tests use high concentrations of the challenge agent, are conducted for long periods of time (up to 312 minutes), and penetration is determined only at the end of the test (giving a time-weighted penetration value). These tests, due to the high concentrations and long durations, can allow the challenge agent to load or fill the spaces between the filter fibers. This is known as filter caking, and it can substantially increase the filter's efficiency and, therefore, lower the penetration. The overall test penetration (which must be no more than 1% to pass the test) may therefore be much less than that which occurred at the beginning of the test.

In the relatively dust-free health care setting, workers exposed to TB patients would need protection from aerosols of approximately 1–5 μm in diameter.[12,56,68] High filter loading should not occur, so the current test methods may underestimate the number of TB droplets penetrating through DM and DFM filters. Several studies have shown, in fact, that these filters have widely varying efficiencies against aerosols measuring less than 2–4 μm.[15,16,38,48] Results from three of these studies are shown in Figures 7, 8, and 9. Figure 7 shows that at 10 liters per minute, DM filter leakage can be as much as 13% (87% efficiency) with a 1-μm particle. This increases to as much as 26% (74% efficiency) at higher flow rates (Fig. 8). This is in sharp contrast to the 99% efficiency required during the certification process. The filter leakage from the DFM respirators tested is less than 1% (Fig. 9) for a 1-μm particle. NIOSH is in the process of revising the certification regulations, which will remove the current testing deficiencies.

Viewed differently, the data also show that some DM and all the tested DFM respirators are efficient at removing particles measuring about 1 μm. The protection provided by a DM respirator against TB aerosols would depend substantially on which brand of respirator was selected. However, filter efficiency decreases with smaller particles, and the precise aerodynamic size distribution of viable, infectious TB droplet nuclei is not well established.

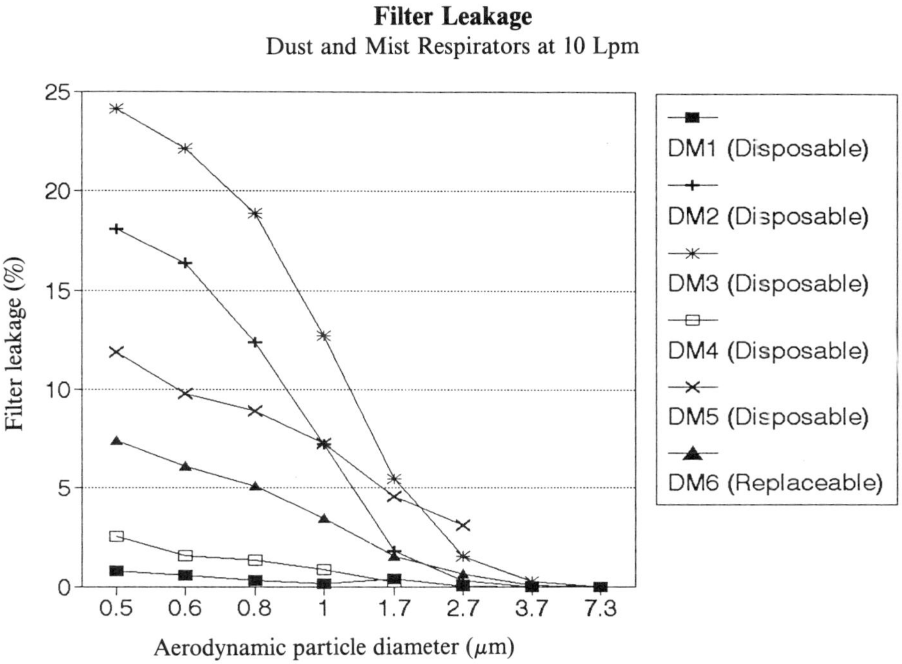

FIGURE 7. Percentage of filter leakage versus aerodynamic particle size for six dust and mist respirators (DM1–DM6) tested at a flow rate of 10 liters per minute. The first five are disposable respirators, and the sixth has replaceable filters.[15,16,38]

Surgical masks have been demonstrated to have even more variability in filter leakage, ranging from 5–100% for 1-μm particles (Fig. 10).[81] This is one of the reasons surgical masks are not recommended for protection against TB. As seen in Figure 10 and in other sources,[79,80] however, some current surgical masks have very efficient filters.

HEPA filters are certified using a very penetrating aerosol (approximately 0.3 μm). The performance standard requires these filters to be at least 99.97% efficient (penetration less than or equal to 0.03%). They are also the only filters certified for use against highly toxic materials.[25] Also, ANSI specifically recommends the use of only high-efficiency filter respirators against aerosols having an aerodynamic size smaller than 2 μm.[6]

Respirator Program

In October 1993, OSHA announced its new policy regarding protection of workers from TB.[63] With regard to personal respiratory protection, this document requires "the use of NIOSH-approved HEPA respirators as a minimum level of respiratory protection when employees perform high hazard procedures, enter isolation rooms housing individuals who may have tuberculosis or transporting such individuals in a closed vehicle. Whenever respirator use is indicated, a complete respirator protection program must be in place." The standard OSHA requirement for a respiratory protection program whenever respirators are used is based on the general industrial hygiene principle that, unless emphasis is carefully

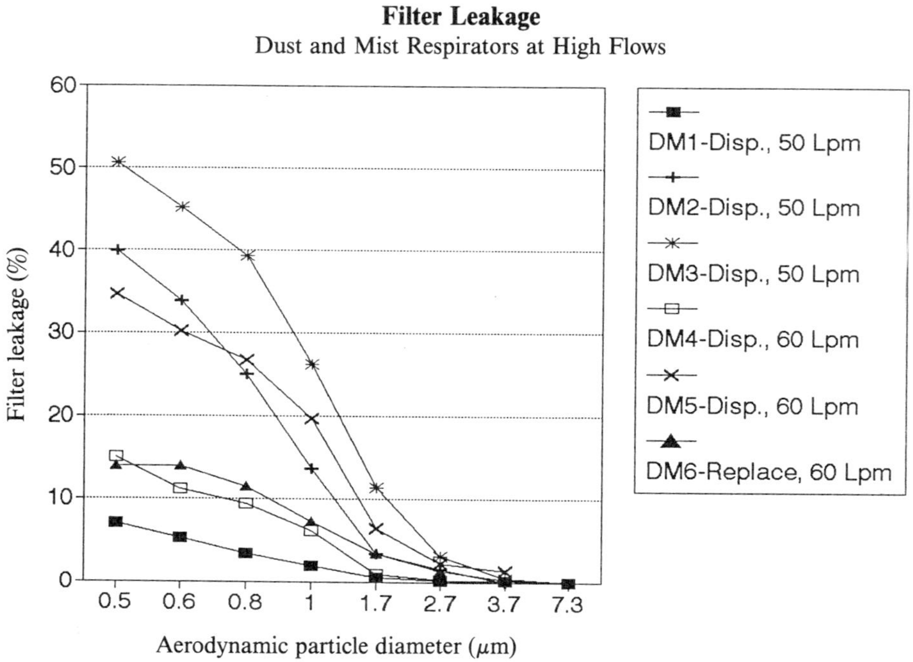

FIGURE 8. Percentage of filter leakage versus aerodynamic particle size for six dust and mist respirators (DM1–DM6) tested at high flow rates. Respirators are the same as in Figure 7.[15,16,38]

placed on a number of details, respirators will not provide the expected protection to workers.[6,12,59]

The OSHA-mandated requirements for a minimal acceptable program are given in 29 CFR 1910.134 (b) and consist of the following:

- Written standard operating procedures
- Selection of respirators based on the hazard
- User instruction and training
- Cleaning and disinfection of the respirators
- Proper storage of the respirators
- Routine inspection of the respirators
- Surveillance of work area conditions
- Evaluation of the respirator protection program
- Medical evaluation of the user's ability to wear a respirator
- The use of certified respirators

It is generally recommended that a respirator program be administered by one person with the technical and professional background necessary to make sound judgments regarding respirator use.

Continuing surveillance of the workplace conditions and worker exposure should be conducted. The purpose of this surveillance is to evaluate the work environment for conditions such as changes in work practices and ventilation that could affect the workers' exposure. The information gathered should be used to help determine if the respiratory protection is effective.

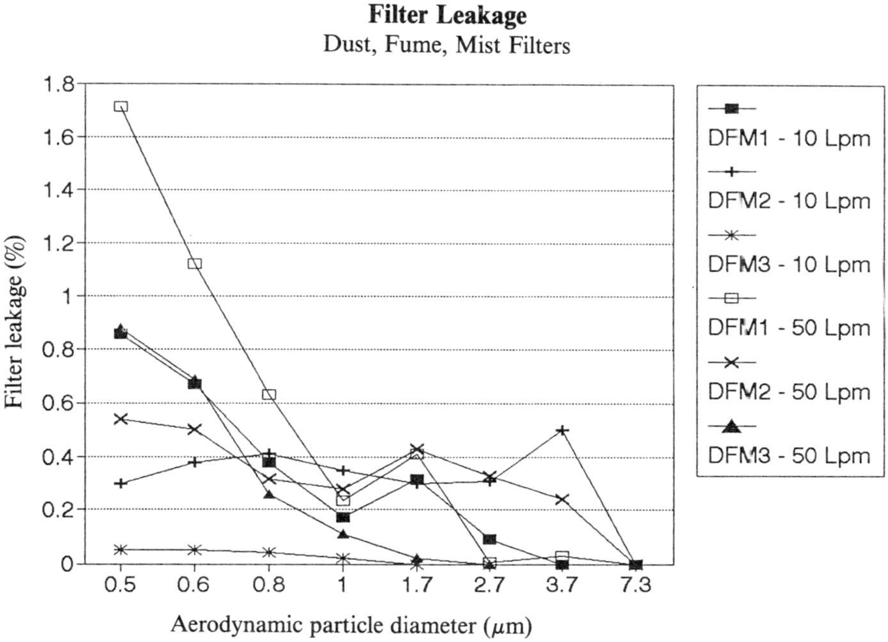

FIGURE 9. Percentage of filter leakage versus aerodynamic particle size for three dust, fume, and mist respirators (DFM1–DFM3) tested at flow rates of both 10 and 50 liters per minute.[15,16,38]

It is generally recommended that the respiratory protection program be evaluated at least once a year,[6] which would logically be a part of a TB infection control program evaluation in health care settings. Frequent evaluation of respirator use will determine if the workers are using the correct respirators and wearing them properly. The workers should be consulted about their acceptance of respirators.

Respirator Fitness Determinations

According to OSHA regulations,[24] persons should not be assigned to tasks requiring the use of respirators unless it has been determined that they are physically able to perform the work and use the respirator. A physician should determine what health and physical conditions are pertinent to this assessment. Although agent-specific OSHA regulations often require certain exams and tests in this evaluation, the generic respirator regulations cited, which would apply to health care workers exposed to TB, do not. It is mandated that the respirator wearer's medical status be reviewed periodically.

These regulations obviously contrast with the traditional absence of any such requirement—other than meeting basic criteria to safely and effectively work—for the use of surgical masks in the health care industry. The American Industrial Hygiene Association,[26] ANSI,[7] and NIOSH[61] have detailed (and different) recommendations on medical surveillance for respirator wear, and several reviews of the various effects of respiratory devices and other recommendations have been published.[10,36,39,49,53,66] Unfortunately, despite these efforts, there still is no

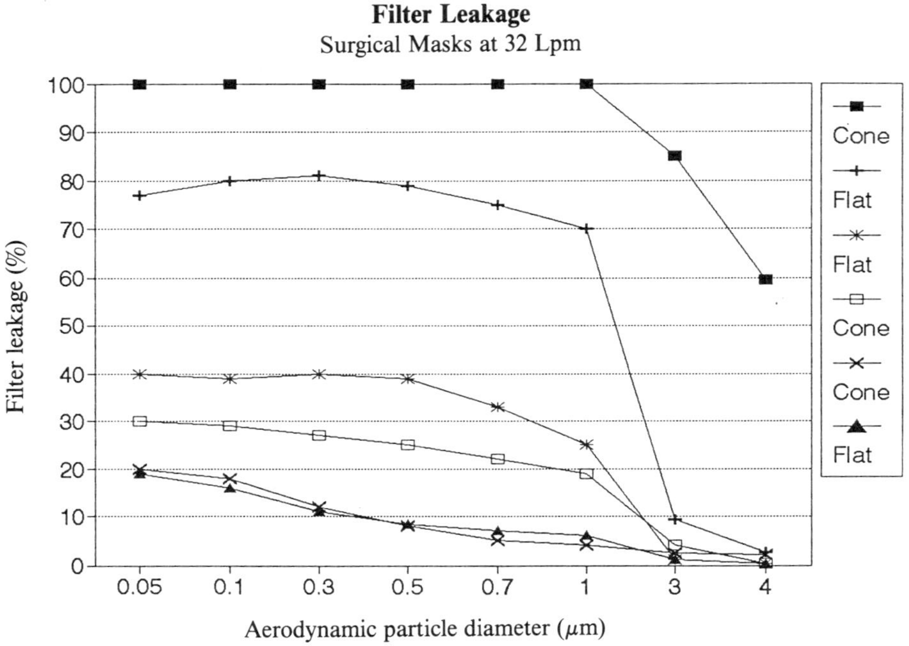

FIGURE 10. Percentage of filter leakage versus aerodynamic particle size for six different surgical masks tested at 32 liters per minute.[81]

standard approach to the evaluation process and decision logic in determining fitness for usage of any given type of device.

In determining the fitness to wear a respirator, NIOSH currently recommends at least a brief history and physical examination, which could be done by paramedicals and does not recommend routine chest x-ray or spirometry.[61] In the health care setting, it would seem reasonable to start with a brief screening medical questionnaire (Fig. 11) that could be used to exempt a large majority of workers from a physical examination or laboratory tests. Although spirometry, recommended by some,[53] is not unreasonable, particularly when the airborne hazard can directly cause pulmonary impairment, it is not likely to detect significant abnormalities missed by the questionnaire. If used, values showing mild impairment[3] would not be expected to preclude safe respirator wear.[36,39,53]

Respirator Fit Test and Fit Check Methods

A fit test is conducted to ensure that a respirator face piece is properly matched to the wearer. It uses a challenge agent to determine the fit of a particular respirator to a particular individual. There are two types of fit tests: qualitative and quantitative. A qualitative fit test is a pass/fail test that relies on the wearer's sensory response (smell, taste, or irritation) to detect the challenge agent. A quantitative fit test uses an instrument to measure the challenge agent inside and outside of the respirator.[59]

Three agents are currently used and accepted by OSHA and the general industrial hygiene community in qualitative fit testing:

Sample Health Care Worker Respirator Questionnaire

1. Have you ever been told by a doctor that you have asthma, chronic bronchitis, emphysema, or other chronic chest condition?
   _____ Yes _____ No
2. Do you have any breathing difficulties with normal work or other usual activities?
   _____ Yes _____ No
3. Have you been told by a doctor that you have angina or other heart abnormalities (including high blood pressure)?
   _____ Yes _____ No
4. Do you have chest pains, skipped heart beats, lightheaded spells, or other symptoms you think are related to your heart?
   _____ Yes _____ No
5. Are you aware of any medical or other reasons that you think would prevent you from safely wearing a respiratory protective device in your work?
   _____ Yes _____ No
6. Has your present or past work involved wearing either a surgical mask or respirator?
   _____ Yes _____ No
7. If the answer to #6 is "Yes," have you had problems that have prevented you from wearing the device as required?
   _____ Yes _____ No

Please explain all "Yes" answers:

Number Explanation

FIGURE 11. A screening questionnaire for determining fitness to wear a respirator for people potentially exposed to tuberculosis.

- Iso-amyl acetate (banana oil), which can be used only with organic vapor cartridges or canisters (or respirators with replaceable filters, which can include the organic vapor type).
- Saccharin, which can be used with DM and DFM as well as HEPA respirators. However, it is not recommended by NIOSH due to its potential carcinogenicity. Its use is allowed by OSHA in certain substance standards.
- Irritant smoke, which can be used only with high-efficiency filter respirators because of its small particle size.

Quantitative fit tests generally use corn oil or sodium chloride as the challenge agent. The detailed protocols for conducting both qualitative and quantitative fit tests can be found in the OSHA Asbestos Standard.[20] In addition, OSHA allows the use of the Portacount™ (TSI, Inc., St. Paul, MN), which measures particulate matter in ambient air, for conducting quantitative fit testing.[71]

If a quantitative fit test is used, ANSI recommends that before using the respirator the wearer should obtain a fit factor at least 10 times greater than the APF of the respirator.[6] If a qualitative fit test is used, it should be designed to assess fit factors 10 times greater than the APF. This arbitrary safety factor is intended to ensure protection during actual use where deterioration in respiratory protection is known to occur. Fit testing is recommended at least once a year and is repeated when a condition develops that may interfere with face piece sealing, such as weight and dental changes.[59]

Qualitative fit tests are usually fast, require no complicated and expensive equipment, and are easily performed in the field. Because they rely on the wearer's subjective response, they may not be entirely reliable. The main advantage of a quantitative fit test is that it does not rely on a subjective response. However, it requires expensive equipment and trained personnel to operate the equipment. In addition, a metal probe usually must be put through the face piece in order to sample the air inside of it. Therefore, the same face piece cannot be used for the fit test and in the workplace. Although present fit tests are somewhat limited, it is likely that additional new challenge aerosols and methods will be developed and validated to test all respirators.

In contrast to the infrequently conducted fit tests, OSHA requires respirator users to perform a fit check each time they don their respirator,[24] which helps ensure that the respirator will give the anticipated level of protection each time it is worn. Fit checks and fit tests have basically the same function: detecting respirator face piece fits that do not provide adequate protection, usually defined as fit factors less than 10 times the APF.

Although OSHA notes that the manufacturer's instructions should be followed in performing a fit check, two standard methods are commonly used. A negative-pressure fit check is carried out by completely closing the pathway of the inhaled air so that it does not pass air; inhaling gently so that the face piece collapses slightly; and holding the breath for 10 seconds. If the face piece remains collapsed and the wearer does not detect any inward leaking air, the respirator face piece seal is probably adequate. A positive-pressure test is similar to the negative-pressure test except that it is the pathway for the exhaled air that is sealed, and the wearer exhales rather than inhales. If the wearer detects a slight positive pressure being built up in the face piece and does not detect outward leakage of air, the fit is considered to be satisfactory.

Both the negative-pressure and the positive-pressure tests can be performed only on respirators using a tight-fitting face piece such as a half mask or full face piece. Most disposable respirators currently cannot easily be fit checked reliably since the entire face piece surface is intended to permit air flow in both directions, and it is difficult to completely cover the mask with one's hands. Manufacturers are developing different methods, such as plastic covers or valve systems, in an effort to allow the wearer to perform a more meaningful fit check with these devices (Fig. 12). Research to validate the usefulness of these new devices is needed.

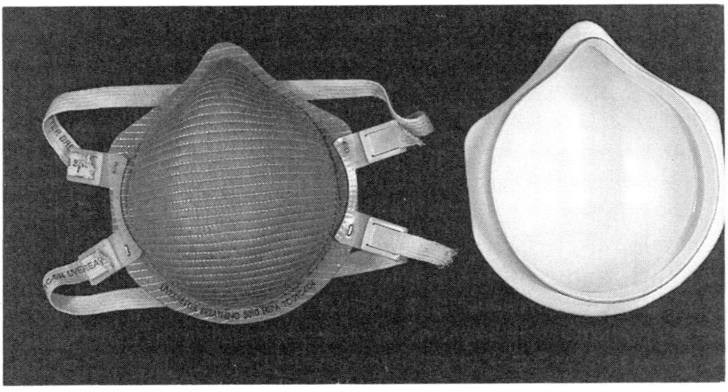

FIGURE 12. Disposable high-efficiency particulate air (HEPA) respirator with plastic fit check cup (right) designed to totally occlude the face piece filter to allow a more meaningful fit check.

TABLE 2. Costs of Various Respirators and Replaceable Filters*

Description	Price Range
Elastomeric half-mask respirator	$19.00–25.00
Replaceable dust, mist filters	$0.68–1.10 each (normally 2 needed per mask)
Replaceable dust, fume, and mist filters	$1.35–2.34 each (normally 2 needed per mask)
Replaceable high-efficiency (HEPA) filters	$1.35–2.34 each (normally 2 needed per mask)
Disposable dust, mist respirator	$0.68–1.08
Disposable dust, fume, and mist respirator	$5.23–8.21
Disposable high-efficiency respirator	$5.23–15.00
Powered air-purifying respirator with high-efficiency filters	$450–600
Replacement powered air-purifying high-efficiency filters	$6.85–9.02 each
Supplied-air respirator (with 100 feet of airline hose)	$1,200–1,525
Self-contained breathing apparatus	$2,400–3,500

* These are retail prices for small quantities. Lower prices may be obtained by ordering direct from the manufacturer in large quantities.

Cost of Respirators

The costs of the various types of respirators are listed in Table 2. The cost of the actual respirator is only part of the cost of the entire respiratory protection program. The medical evaluation, fit testing, maintenance program, and the other components contribute significantly to the required expertise and cost of a respiratory protection program.

Respiratory Feasibility: Special Considerations

When selecting a respirator to provide protection against TB, certain feasibility issues and special considerations must be addressed. In the health care setting, the impact of respirator use on patient care must be considered. All respirators impair voice communications to some degree. Those made of heavier materials such as silicone rubber cause even more speech impairment, although voice diaphragms alleviate this problem to some extent. Elastomeric face pieces, especially the larger and typically dark ones, may present an "intimidating" appearance to patients accustomed to the smaller, light-colored surgical masks commonly used in health care settings. In this regard, disposable particulate respirators more closely resemble surgical masks and may not be as intimidating.

Virtually all respirators will be perceived as less comfortable than surgical masks in the health care community. This may relate to the tighter fit of these devices required for adequate protection, an increase in breathing resistance, and an increased weight in some cases. Particularly during initial experience, these factors will lead to increased stress for many users. In some industrial settings, powered air-purifying respirators (PAPRs), with their cooling airflow, may be perceived as more comfortable.

The more protective respirators, including PAPRs and atmosphere-supplying respirators, have several disadvantages that relate to their complex design and increased size or weight. These factors could reduce the health care worker's ability to deliver patient care efficiently and in some cases could present increased safety risks. For example, PAPRs generate some background noise due to the blower and to air being forced into the face piece, which may impair auscultation and understanding of speech. The battery assembly is somewhat bulky and must be recharged for at least 8 hours after each 8 hours of use. The advantages and disadvantages of the various respirator types are described in Table 3.

RESPIRATORY PROTECTION APPLIED TO TUBERCULOSIS

A number of issues have been raised regarding the use of respirators for protection against TB. The first and fundamental issue is the need for and efficacy

TABLE 3. Advantages and Disadvantages of Various Types of Respirators

Type of Respirator	Advantages	Disadvantages/Limitations
Particulate, nonpowered	Light weight Small size Ease of maintenance Little physiologic stress to wearer Mobility is not restricted Simple design—easily understood by wearer *HEPA filters* Do not degrade with high humidities or oil mists *Disposable respirators* Require no maintenance, cleaning or disinfecting Low breathing resistance	Negative pressure may allow leakage particularly if not fitted properly Facial hair or scars may interfere with face seal *Dust and mist and dust, fume, and mist respirators* May degrade if not stored properly or if used in atmospheres containing high humidity or oil mists *Disposable respirators* Measuring facial fit in the field may be difficult
Powered air-purifying respirators	Decreased inhalation resistance may make respirator more comfortable to wear Mobility is not restricted *Loose-fitting* No large sealing surfaces on the face allows some people (i.e., ones with facial scars or facial hair) to achieve an adequate fit	Weight and bulk may make respirator more difficult to wear than non-powered respirators Complex and continual maintenance Airflow and blower will create noise that will hamper wearer's ability to hear Elastomeric face piece and blower noise make clear speech difficult
Type C airline respirators	Low breathing resistance Light weight and low bulk Long duration *Positive-pressure respirators* Higher protection afforded to wearer *Loose-fitting* No large sealing surfaces on the face allows some (i.e., ones with facial scars or facial hair) to achieve an adequate fit	Cutting, crushing or kinking of hose will lead to complete loss of respiratory protection* Restricts mobility Requires independent source of Grade D breathing air Complex maintenance *Loose fitting* Continuous airflow will create noise that will hamper wearer's ability to hear
Self-contained breathing apparatus (SCBA)	Mobility is not restricted *Positive pressure respirators* Highest protection of all respirators	Bulk and weight make them unsuitable for strenuous work or in constricted space Limited service life Complex maintenance Complex design requires more training for wearer and maintenance staff

*A combination supplied-air/SCBA will eliminate this disadvantage.

of respiratory protection as a necessary part of the protection hierarchy. Surgical masks were recommended by the American Thoracic Society and CDC prior to 1990[1,83] and have been in use at least since the 1930s,[9] when the initial U.S. public health TB programs were developed. However, most TB prevention programs in health care settings involve multiple safeguards, and the specific need for, or effectiveness of, surgical masks has not been clearly shown. Indeed, given the often loose-fitting type of masks used particularly in past years, one might not have expected much benefit from this protection. Accordingly, some physicians in the past and currently have not worn any mask while in TB isolation rooms.

Traditionally, more emphasis has been placed on early detection and isolation and covering the patient's mouth during coughing or sneezing to prevent or reduce the generation of infectious aerosols.[1,2,8,12,60,68,69,83] While these measures must remain as the cornerstone of prevention, required close contact with a coughing patient, particularly when covering the mouth is not possible or tolerated, necessitates personal respiratory protection in addition to other measures. Reports of multiple infections following certain cough-inducing or other aerosol-generating procedures support this practice.[51,57] A high level of respiratory protection would especially be needed for health care workers with immunosuppression and in facilities where other infection-control practices are inadequate.[31] The spread of the human immunodeficiency virus and the emergence of multidrug-resistant strains of TB have also increased the number and duration of TB patient exposures for many health care workers.[40]

If one accepts that personal respiratory protection against TB is needed in certain circumstances, a vital second issue is which type is appropriate. Here lies the main present debate, which is complicated by a lack of data and the application of much theoretical information. Several aspects of the discussion are noted below and in the next section.

A third issue relates to whether bioaerosols behave differently from nonbiologic aerosols in terms of filter penetration. Unfortunately, data are lacking in this area. However, it is well known that filter penetration depends on filter characteristics, filter loading (the amount of contaminant occluding the filter), the size distribution of the particulates, the air flow through the filter, and electrostatic charges on the filter and particulates in the aerosol.[42,49] Unless the biologic aerosol were able to actively degrade the filter media, one would not expect it to behave differently from a nonbiological aerosol with the same physical characteristics. Data from the U.S. Army comparing filter penetration of *Bacillus subtilis* spores to similarly sized corn oil aerosols found very similar results, supporting this view,[77] although the round spores might not be considered the best surrogate for TB organisms. However, recent data have shown that *Mycobacterium chelonei* aerosols have very similar penetration characteristics as the same aerodynamically sized (0.8 μm) latex particles when tested against one surgical mask and selected DM, DFM, and HEPA respirators.[18]

A fourth issue is that of the particle size distribution of TB aerosols, which is important since DM and DFM respirators are not considered to reliably filter out particles smaller than 2 μm in aerodynamic diameter.[6,60] Again, published data with TB using modern assays are virtually nonexistent. It is generally accepted that the TB organism itself varies from 0.2–0.6 μm in width and 0.5–4.0 μm in length.[72,74] However, the droplet nuclei arising from infectious TB patients are thought to be about 1–5 μm.[12,56,68] One study showed approximately 25% of droplets expulsed from the respiratory tract of normal volunteers to be smaller than 3 μm.[50] Recent work demonstrates that some mycobacteria can exist in viable form in aerosols of approximately 1 μm in diameter.[18] Better data are needed, which should include the important aspects of the viability and infectivity as well as the number of particles in the various TB droplet nuclei size fractions.

The reuse of "disposable" respirators in the health care setting is another issue, in part brought on by the added expense of most respirators compared to surgical masks. In many industrial settings, the high dust exposures eventually occlude the filter, causing unacceptable breathing resistance, which requires replacement of the respirator or filter, often after a day's use. This is not the case in health care settings, and reuse for several weeks may be possible. However, this reuse may create problems with logistics and safe temporary storage of the respirators. In addition, it is not known when and if contamination by various organisms prevalent in the health care setting would indicate the need for replacement. Local infection control experts will likely be expected to evaluate and make recommendations in this regard.

EXISTING RECOMMENDATIONS AND RATIONALES

Table 4 presents six recent recommendations regarding the use of respiratory protective devices for workers exposed to TB aerosols. A brief rationale for each recommendation is given below.

The familiar surgical mask recommendation has been in place for many years.[1,83] The basis for this recommendation is (1) the long-standing standard of care in which surgical masks are used to prevent the expulsion of infectious materials from the wearer's mouth and nose in operating rooms, (2) the logical step that the same mask would prevent the inhalation by the wearer of at least some airborne particles, and (3) the knowledge that usually several months of TB exposure are needed before most individuals become infected.[67,68]

Although there are no good data to determine the effectiveness or the health costs (in terms of TB infections, adverse reactions to isoniazid, and clinical TB) of this surgical mask policy, the logarithmically declining TB rate in this country from 1955–1985 did not suggest a major deficiency. However, because of inadequate TB surveillance in many health care settings, one cannot assume that TB transmission has not occurred in these settings.[41] Still, some experts would prefer

TABLE 4. Tuberculosis Personal Respiratory Protection Recommendations

Recommendation	Date	Source
Surgical mask	Before 1990	ATS/CDC[1]
Disposable particulate respirator (includes DM, DFM, and HEPA respirators)	December 1990	CDC[12]
Dust, fume, and mist respirator	May 1992	OSHA Region II[62]
Powered air-purifying respirator/positive-pressure airline	September 1992	NIOSH[60]
Performance criteria (currently leading to a HEPA respirator)	October 1993	CDC (revised draft)[13]
HEPA respirator	October 1993	Federal OSHA[63]

DM = dust, mist respirator; DFM = dust, fume, and mist respirator; HEPA = high-efficiency particulate air (also called high-efficiency) respirator; ATS = American Thoracic Society; CDC = Centers for Disease Control; OSHA = Occupational Safety and Health Administration; NIOSH = National Institute for Occupational Safety and Health.

to see evidence of the failure of surgical masks in the setting of a properly operated TB infection control program before changing to new and more expensive devices.[75]

Individual hospital "epidemics" of TB, involving workers as well as patients, are generally thought to reflect multiple failures in the public health approach to TB control.[8,31] They have led to a reevaluation of all measures used in the past, including respiratory protective devices. The first change in recommendations regarding respiratory protective devices came with 1990 CDC guidelines[12] that recommended disposable particulate respirators (PR) as better designed and more effective in protecting workers from TB aerosols and that noted the deficiencies of surgical masks. PRs include dust and mist (DM), dust, fume, and mist (DFM), and high-efficiency particulate air (HEPA) air-purifying masks, with protection and cost increasing respectively. The CDC document *recommended* that a respiratory program be included with the use of particulate respirators. (It is not clear to what extent all authors and subsequent users realized that the use of a respirator versus a surgical mask would necessarily be accompanied by OSHA enforcement requirements.)

Supporters of the 1990 CDC guidelines cite preliminary data suggesting hospital TB epidemics become controlled when the guidelines were followed, sometimes even without change in traditional personal respiratory protection.[52,73,82] In collaboration with other groups, the American Thoracic Society also has written a statement on TB control[2] that substantially agrees with the CDC guidelines. This joint statement by CDC, ATS, American Academy of Pediatrics, and Infectious Disease Society of America specifically recomments a disposable particulate respirator in circumstances when personal respiratory protection is needed.[2]

DFM respirators, which were recommended by OSHA Region II,[62] are tested with a smaller particle aerosol (lead fume) in addition to the silica test used for DM devices. Unlike DM respirators, DFM devices also are qualitatively fit tested on a panel of 10 subjects who are selected to represent a variety of facial sizes in the NIOSH certification process. They should therefore provide better protection against TB aerosols, as available data predict (*see* Fig. 7–9).[16,17,38]

Guidelines published by NIOSH in 1992[60] recommend only the most protective filter (HEPA). The recommendation is based on uncertainties of the particle size distribution of TB aerosols and the potentially lethal outcome if a respirator fails. In addition, the guidelines recognized a serious problem with any nonpowered air-purifying respirator: Regardless of the filter efficiency, 10% or more face seal leakage can occur with half-mask devices. Because of this, for moderate TB exposures, NIOSH recommended a PAPR with a HEPA filter, because it will create, under most work conditions, a slightly positive pressure in the face piece. Therefore, any face seal leakage will tend to be outward rather than inward.

For high-exposure settings, such as during intubation or bronchoscopy of a TB patient, NIOSH recommended a positive-pressure air-line respirator with a tight-fitting half-mask. This device is designed to maintain a greater and more consistent positive pressure in the face piece versus the PAPR; it also uses an independent pure air source to avoid filter leakage problems. The rationale for this recommendation was that for higher exposures, a higher level of expected protection is needed. The NIOSH recommendations were stated as minimum acceptable respirators, and it was noted that no respirator may provide complete protection from an airborne hazard.

In May 1994, NIOSH changed its policy, stating it was in the process of revising its recommendations for respirators for use against tuberculosis. It stated that it was currently endorsing the recommendations in the draft CDC guidelines.[59a]

The draft revised CDC recommendations[13] published in October 1993 are meant to represent a compromise between the need to provide the best protection to the worker and the need for workers to be able to deliver competent health care. It is expected that, in the final version, the respirator criteria listed will be essentially unchanged but that better justification will be given. Instead of recommending a specific type of current respirator, performance guidelines are stated in the hope of stimulating cost-effective improvements in design and specific evaluations related to TB. These criteria are:

1. Ninety-five percent filter efficiency of 1-μm particles at flow rates up to 50 Lpm. (The choice of 95% filter efficiency is not explained in the document.)
2. Ability to perform a reliable qualitative or quantitative fit test, yielding no more than 10% face seal leakage for most workers
3. Ability to fit different face sizes and having at least three respirator sizes
4. Ability to be fit checked

The only respirators that are currently certified by NIOSH to meet these criteria are HEPA respirators. However, new filter certification regulations being developed by NIOSH would replace the DM, DFM, and HEPA filters with three new types of filters, all of which would be tested with the most penetrating aerosol size (approximately 0.3 μm). The three filters, to be called type A, B, and C, will have 99.97%, 99%, and 95% efficiency, respectively. All three of these proposed types would meet the draft CDC criteria. The final rule for these new filter certifications is expected to be published in the *Federal Register* in December 1994.

Several earlier versions of the CDC recommendations have been discussed in the literature. In one, "protective" surgical masks (those sold to provide protection to the wearer, as from laser plumes) were suggested as the minimal TB protection.[4] However, the lack of a formal uniform certification process and remaining concerns regarding face fit reduced the viability of this concept.

The federal OSHA mandatory guidelines[63] of October 1993 include the use of HEPA respirators in selected TB exposure situations. The rationale includes the fact that because no known safe exposure level exists for TB, one should select respirators with a minimal margin of error. Also noted were the concerns described earlier regarding deficiencies in the present certification tests of DM and DFM respirators and the resultant lack of assurance that these respirators would remove TB droplet nuclei. Because PAPRs may interfere with patient care or could be infeasible for other reasons, they were not required.

The October 1993 federal OSHA TB enforcement guidance is based on its general duty clause.[63] OSHA has begun to conduct formal rulemaking on this issue and plans to have a proposed rule published by the spring of 1995. As of October 1994, it is unknown whether OSHA intends to adopt the CDC guidelines with regard to required personal respiratory protection; to do so would bring all three federal organizations (OSHA, CDC, and NIOSH) into agreement.

Additional new recommendations regarding respiratory protection have been or are being developed by several other organizations, including the Joint Commission on Accreditation of Healthcare Organizations (regarding TB exposure),[45] the American National Standards Institute (regarding bioaerosols), and the American Thoracic Society (on respiratory protection guidelines).

CONCLUSIONS

The role of respiratory protective devices in the prevention of tuberculosis has not changed significantly in the last few years; the devices are still used to provide additional protection in limited circumstances in which other controls may not be effective. However, the recommended type of device, unchallenged for more than half a century, now includes a wide variety of devices, with differing degrees of predicted protection, substantially differing costs, and associated practices new to the health care community. Recent federal OSHA enforcement policy has mandated the use of HEPA respirators and an associated respiratory program for the protection of workers against TB in selected exposure settings.[63]

No conclusive evidence exists to show the effectiveness of any of these devices in the clinical setting against TB, but a large body of data indicates true and significant differences in afforded protection among the various types of personal respiratory protection devices. It would thus seem that a major issue is not the greater protection provided by the newly recommended devices, but rather how much personal respiratory protection is needed in the variety of TB exposure settings and for the variety of workers across the country. This issue must be correlated with the worker's ability to deliver safe and adequate health care to patients.

Additional conclusions include the following:

1. The role of respiratory protective devices is secondary to other, general measures in the prevention of the spread of TB.

2. Even when these other measures are in place, there will still be circumstances, such as close contact with a coughing, infectious patient, that will require effective respiratory protective devices for adequate protection against TB.

3. Many current surgical masks are not thought to provide a good face seal and often come in only one size.

4. Data indicate that there is a very large variability in filter efficiency, particularly among different brands of surgical masks but also among dust, mist respirators.

5. HEPA respirators provide consistent and very high filter efficiency and can be quantitatively fit tested with commercially available kits. At least some disposable HEPA respirators have been designed to be fit checked in a more meaningful way, although proof of their effectiveness is needed.

6. Masking of the infectious TB patient is still considered an effective source control by most experts.[12,13,68,69] Since the explosive force of coughing or sneezing may break the seal of most devices, it is not known if certified respirators are more effective than surgical masks for this purpose. Obviously, respirators with exhalation valves would not be appropriate for this use.

7. Although many workers will find respirators uncomfortable, the small physiologic burden of most respirators should be adequately tolerated by most health care workers. Minimal medical screening should be adequate to ensure worker safety and to detect workers who will need closer evaluation.

8. One of the major problems with respiratory protective devices is face seal leakage. To the extent that respiratory protective devices are needed for adequate protection, it is important to minimize this problem. The standard industrial hygiene approach is to have multiple styles and sizes of respirators, perform fit tests, and do fit checks before each respirator use.

9. Much empirical information is needed to allow better assessment of the need for, selection of, and proper use of respiratory protective devices against TB.

10. It seems likely that improvements in respiratory protective devices will increase acceptance by both workers and patients while maintaining adequate protection from TB. Improvements in certification should assist in this advancement.

11. No respiratory protective device will provide complete protection. Workers' understanding of this and all aspects of TB control should aid in the effort to prevent TB spread in health care settings.

REFERENCES

1. American Thoracic Society: Control of tuberculosis. Am Rev Respir Dis 128:336–342, 1983.
2. American Thoracic Society: Control of tuberculosis in the United States. Am Rev Respir Dis 146:1623–1633, 1992.
3. American Thoracic Society: Lung function testing: Selection of reference values and interpretative strategies. Am Rev Respir Dis 144:1202–1218, 1991.
4. Anonymous: CDC draft guidelines for TB renew infection control debate. Hosp Epidemiol Infect Control 43:36–39, 1993.
5. ANSI Z88.2-1969: American National Standard for Respiratory Protection. New York, American National Standards Institute, 1969.
6. ANSI Z88.2-1992: American National Standard for Respiratory Protection. New York, American National Standards Institute, 1992.
7. ANSI Z88.6-1984: American National Standard for Respirator Protection-Respirator Use—Physical Qualifications for Personnel. New York, American National Standards Institute, 1984.
8. Barnes PF, Barrows SA: Tuberculosis in the 1990s. Ann Intern Med 119:400–410, 1993.
9. Beck WC: The surgical mask: Another 'sacred cow'? AORN J 55:955–957, 1992.
10. Beckett WS: Certifying the worker for respirator use. Semin Occup Med 1:119–124, 1986.
11. Bentley RA, Bostock GJ, Longson DJ, Roff MW: Determination of the quantitative fit factors of various types of respiratory protective equipment. J Int Soc Respir Prot 2:313–337, 1984.
12. Centers for Disease Control: Guidelines for preventing the transmission of tuberculosis in health-care settings, with special focus on HIV-related disease. MMWR 39(RR-17):1–28, 1990.
13. Centers for Disease Control and Prevention: Draft guidelines for preventing the transmission of tuberculosis in health care facilities, 2nd ed; Notice of comment period. Federal Register 58:52810–52854, October 12, 1993.
14. Charney W, Fisher J, Ishaida C: The inefficiency of surgical masks for protection against droplet nuclei tuberculosis [letter]. J Occup Med 33:943–944, 1991.
15. Chen CC, Lethimäki M, Willeke K: Aerosol penetration through filtering facepieces and respirator cartridges. Am Ind Hyg Assoc J 53:566–574, 1992.
16. Chen CC, Ruuskannen J, Pilacinski W, Willeke K: Filter and leak penetration characteristics of a dust and mist filtering facepiece. Am Ind Hyg J 51:632–639, 1990.
17. Chen CC, Willeke K: Aerosol penetration through surgical masks. Am J Infect Control 20:177–184, 1992.
18. Chen S, Vesley D, Brousseau LM, Vincent JH: Evaluation of single-use masks and respirators for protection of health care workers against mycobacterial aerosols. Am J Infect Control 22:65–74, 1994.
19. Code of Federal Regulations: 21 CFR 878.4040 (Surgical apparel). Washington, DC, US Government Printing Office, Office of the Federal Register, 1993.
20. Code of Federal Regulations: 29 CFR 1910.1001 (Asbestos, tremolite, anthophyllite, and actinolite). Washington, DC, US Government Printing Office, Office of the Federal Register, 1993.
21. Code of Federal Regulations: 29 CFR 1910.1025 (Lead). Washington, DC, US Government Printing Office, Office of the Federal Register, 1993.
22. Code of Federal Regulations: 29 CFR 1910.1027 (Cadmium). Washington, DC, US Government Printing Office, Office of the Federal Register, 1993.
23. Code of Federal Regulations: 29 CFR 1910.1043 (Cotton Dust). Washington, DC, US Government Printing Office, Office of the Federal Register, 1993.
24. Code of Federal Regulations: 29 CFR 1910.134 (Respiratory protection). Washington, DC, US Government Printing Office, Office of the Federal Register, 1993.
25. Code of Federal Regulations: 30 (Mineral Resources) CFR 11, Respiratory Protective Devices; Tests for permissibility; Fees. Washington, DC, US Government Printing Office, Office of the Federal Register, 1993.

26. Colton CD, Birkner LR, Brousseau LM: Respiratory Protection: A Manual and Guideline, 2nd ed. Akron, American Industrial Hygiene Association, 1991.
27. Colton CE, Johnston AR, Mullins HE, Rhoe CR: Respirator workplace protection factor study on a half-mask dust/mist respirator. Presented at the American Industrial Hygiene Conference, Orlando, May 17, 1990.
28. Davis WT: Filtration efficiency of surgical face masks: The need for more meaningful standards. Am J Infect Control 19:16–18, 1991.
29. Dixon SW, Nelson TJ: Workplace protection factors for negative pressure half-mask facepiece respirators. J Int Soc Respir Prot 2:347–361, 1984.
30. Crutchfield CD, Van Ert MD: An examination of issues affecting the current state of quantitative respirator fit testing. J Int Soc Respir Prot 11:5–18, 1993.
31. Dooley SW, Jarvis WR, Martone WJ, Snider DE: Multidrug-resistant tuberculosis [editorial]. Ann Intern Med 117:257–259, 1992.
32. Gosselink DW, Wilmes DP, Mullins HE: Workplace protection factor study for airborne asbetos. Presented at the American Industrial Hygiene Conference, Dallas, Texas, May 18–23, 1986.
33. Greene VW, Vesley D: Method for evaluating effectiveness of surgical masks. J Bacteriol 83:663–667, 1961.
34. Guy HP: Respirator performance terminology. Am Ind Hyg Assoc J 46:B22–24, 1985.
35. Ha'eri GB, Wiley AM: The efficacy of standard surgical face masks: An investigation using "tracer particles." Clin Orthop 148:160–162, 1980.
36. Harber P: Medical evaluation for respirator use. J Occup Med 26:496–502, 1984.
37. Hinds WC: Aerosol Technology. New York, John Wiley & Sons, 1982.
38. Hinds WC, Kraske G: Performance of dust respirators with facial seal leaks: I. Experimental. Am Ind Hyg Assoc J 48:836–841, 1987.
39. Hodous TK: Screening prospective workers for the ability to use respirators. J Occup Med 28:1074–1080, 1986.
40. Hopewell PC: Impact of human immunodeficiency virus infection on the epidemiology, clinical features, management, and control of tuberculosis. Clin Infect Dis 15:540–547, 1992.
41. Hutton MD, Polder JA: Guidelines for preventing tuberculosis transmission in health care settings: What's new? Am J Infect Control 20:24–26, 1992.
42. Hyatt EC: Respiratory studies for the National Institute for Occupational Safety and Health—July 1, 1972 through June 3, 1973. Los Alamos, NM, Los Alamos Scientific Laboratory, May 1974, Progress Report LA-5620-PR.
43. Hyatt EC: Respirator protection factors. Los Alamos, NM, Los Alamos Scientific Laboratory, Informal Report LA-6084-MS, January 1976.
44. Johnston AR, Myers WR, Colton CE, et al: Review of respirator performance testing in the workplace: Issues and concerns. Am Ind Hyg Assoc J 53:705–712, 1992.
45. Joint Commission on Accreditation of Healthcare Organizations: Controlling occupational exposures to tuberculosis. Number 1. Oakbrook Terrace, IL, Joint Commission of Accreditation of Healthcare Organizations, 1993.
46. Lenhart SW, Campbell DL: Assigned protection factors for two respirator types based on workplace performance testing. Ann Occup Hyg 38:173–182, 1984.
47. Linauskas SH, Kalos F: Study of efficiency and current use of respiratory protective devices. Report prepared for the Atomic Energy Control Board. Ottawa, Canada. Atomic Energy of Canada Limited, 1984.
48. Liu BYH, Fardi B: A fundamental study of respiratory air filtration. Final report for NIOSH Grant #R01 OH01485-01A1, University of Minnesota, Particle Technology Laboratory Publication 680, Minneapolis, 1988.
49. Louhevaara VA: Physiological effects associated with the use of respiratory protective devices: A review. Scand J Work Environ Health 10:275–281, 1984.
50. Loudon RG, Roberts RM: Droplet expulsion from the respiratory tract. Am Rev Respir Dis 95:435–442, 1967.
51. Malasky C, Jordan T, Potulski F, Reichman LB: Occupational tuberculous infections among pulmonary physicians in training. Am Rev Respir Dis 142:505–507, 1990.
52. Maloney S, Pearson M, Gordon M, et al: Evaluation of recommended infection control measures in preventing nosocomial transmission of multidrug-resistant tuberculosis [abstract]. Proceedings of third annual meeting of the Society for Hospital Epidemiology of America. Chicago, April 18–20, 1993.
53. Mayo Pulmonary Services: Respirator clearance exams include spirometry. Airflow Update 3(6):1, 1988.

54. Myers WR, Peach MJ III, Allender J: Workplace protection factor measurements on powered air-purifying respirators at a secondary lead smelter—test protocol. Am Ind Hyg Assoc J 45:236–241, 1984.
55. Myers WR, Peach MJ III, Cutright K, Iskander W: Workplace protection factor measurements on powered air-purifying respirators at a secondary lead smelter—results and discussion. Am Ind Hyg Assoc J 45:681–688, 1984.
56. Nardell EA: Dodging droplet nuclei. Am Rev Respir Dis 142:501–503, 1990.
57. Nardell EA, Keegan J, Cheney SA, Etkind SC: Airborne infection—theoretical limits of protection achievable by building ventilation. Am Rev Respir Dis 144:302–306, 1991.
58. NIOSH Guide to Industrial Respiratory Protection. Cincinnati, NIOSH 1976, US Dept of Health, Education and Welfare publication NIOSH 76-189.
59. NIOSH Guide to Industrial Respiratory Protection. Cincinnati, NIOSH 1987, US Dept of Health and Human Services publication NIOSH 87-116.
59a. NIOSH internal communication, May 16, 1994.
60. NIOSH Recommended Guidelines for Personal Respiratory Protection of Workers in Health-Care Facilities Potentially Exposed to Tuberculosis. Atlanta, National Institute for Occupational Safety and Health, 1992.
61. NIOSH Respirator Decision Logic. Cincinnati, NIOSH, 1987, US Dept of Health and Human Services publication 87-108.
62. Occupational Safety and Health Administration, Region II: Compliance guidelines for respiratory protection against tuberculosis. OSHA, Region II, May 1993.
63. Occupational Safety and Health Administration: Enforcement policy and procedures for occupational exposure to tuberculosis. Washington, DC, OSHA, October 20, 1993.
64. Pippin J: Efficiency of face masks in preventing inhalation of airborne contaminants. J Oral Maxillofac Surg 45:319–323, 1987.
65. Plog BA (ed): Fundamentals of Industrial Hygiene. 3rd ed. Chicago, National Safety Council, 1988.
66. Raven PB, Dodson AT, Davis TO: The physiological consequences of wearing industrial respirators: A review. Am Ind Hyg Assoc J 40:517–534, 1979.
67. Riley RL: The hazard is relative. Am Rev Respir Dis 96:623–625, 1967.
68. Riley RL: Airborne infection. Am J Med 57:466–475, 1974.
69. Riley RL, O'Grady F: Airborne infection—transmission and control. New York, Macmillan, 1961.
70. da Roza RA, Cadena-Fix CA, Kramer JE: Powered air-purifying respirator study final report. Livermore, CA, 1986, Lawrence Livermore National Laboratory, University of California, 1986, UCRL-53757.
71. Shepich TJ, Baier E: Memorandum for regional administrators on portacount fit testing device. Washington. DC, US Dept of Labor, Occupational Safety and Health Administration, 1993. OSHA Regulations, Documents, and Technical Information, OSHA CD-ROM (OSHA a93-3).
72. Sherris JC (ed): Medical Microbiology. 2nd ed. New York, Elsevier Science Publishing, 1990.
73. Skaggs BJ, Loibl JM, Carter KD, Hyatt EC: Effects of temperature and humidity on respirator fit under simulated work conditions. Los Alamos, NM, Los Alamos National Laboratory, July 1988, NUREG/CR-5090, LA-11236.
74. Smith D: Mycobacterium tuberculosis and tuberculosis. In Joklik WK, Smith DT (eds): Zinsser Microbiology. 15th ed. New York, Ashton-Century-Crofts, 1972, pp 547–582.
75. Stroud L, Tokars J, Grieco M, et al: Interruption of nosocomial transmission of multidrug-resistant Mycobacterium tuberculosis (MDR-TB) among AIDS patients in a New York City hospital [abstract]. Proceedings of third annual meeting of the Society for Hospital Epidemiology of America, Chicago, April 18–20, 1993.
76. Tuomi T: Face seal leakage of half-masks and surgical masks. Am Ind Hyg Assoc J 46:308–312, 1985.
77. Underwood MA: Commentary from the APIC Guidelines Committee on the Centers for Disease Control "Guidelines for preventing the transmission of tuberculosis in health-care settings, with special focus on HIV-related issues." Am J Infect Control 20:27–29, 1992.
78. U.S. Army Dugway Proving Ground: Final Report: Development test II (PQT-G) of XM40 series protective masks, hoods, and accessories (Contract DAAD-10-81-C-0001). Prepared for U.S. Army Test and Evaluation Command, Aberdeen Proving Ground, MD, January 1988.
79. Vesley D, Langholtz AC, Lauer JL: Clinical implications of surgical mask retention efficiencies for viable and total particles. Infect Surg 2:531–536, 1983.
80. Wadsworth LC, Davis WT: A rapid latex filtration efficiency test method for simulating bacterial filtration efficiency. Particulate and Microbial Control Industry (May/June) 32–37, 1983.

81. Weber A, Willeke K, Marchioni R, et al: Aerosol penetration and leakage characteristics of masks used in the health care industry. Am J Infect Control 21:167–173, 1993.
82. Wenger P, Beck-Sague C, Otten J, et al: Efficacy of control measures in preventing nosocomial transmission of multidrug-resistant Mycobacterium tuberculosis among patients and health care workers [abstract]. Proceedings of the third annual meeting of the Society for Hospital Epidemiology of America. Chicago, April 18–20, 1993.
83. Williams WW: CDC guideline for infection control in hospital personnel Infect Control 4(suppl):328–349, 1983.

JAMIE COHEN, BS
LAURA KENNY, MPH

TUBERCULOSIS IN THE WORKPLACE: A LABOR PERSPECTIVE

From the Health and Safety Department
Service Employees International Union
Washington, DC (JC)
and
New York, New York (LK)

Reprint requests to:
Jamie Cohen
Health and Safety Department
Service Employees International Union
1313 L Street, NW
Washington, DC 20005

On October 22, 1992, the Centers for Disease Control and Prevention (CDC) held an open meeting to review and assess the need to revise the 1990 CDC guidelines for reducing the risk of tuberculosis transmission in health care settings. The interest in this meeting was substantially heightened by the fact that the National Institute for Occupational Safety and Health had recently released its *NIOSH Recommended Guidelines for Personal Respiratory Protection of Workers in Health-Care Facilities Potentially Exposed to Tuberculosis.*[3] The NIOSH guidelines, which explicitly state that "any TB infection due to occupational transmission to workers in health-care facilities is unacceptable" and that NIOSH must "develop criteria . . . which will describe exposure levels . . . at which no worker will suffer impaired health . . . or diminished life expectancy as a result of his [or her] work experience," were greeted by the health care industry with overt hostility. It has long been held in the health care industry that illness and injury are simply part of the job. Labor unions have responded that the application of occupational health principles to other industries has successfully reduced workplace injuries and illnesses dramatically.

Many of the individuals and organizations represented at the meeting objected to the NIOSH recommendation that under certain high risk conditions, a powered, air-purification respirator (PAPR) should be used to protect workers. This respirator, which is most often used in heavy industry, had no role in a health care facility, according to this view. The recommendation to use PAPRs was attacked as "unscientific," "unrealistic," "a diversion of scarce resources," possibly frightening to patients, hazardous to patients and workers, difficult to monitor, and giving health care workers an inappropriate feeling of security that could lead to complacency toward the CDC guidelines.

It was at this meeting that two divergent approaches to illness and injury in the health care setting became apparent. The health care industry has thrived for many years without the constraint of occupational safety and health regulations and supervision common to almost every other industry, but the legitimacy of this laissez faire system was being seriously questioned.

RESISTANCE TO REGULATION IN THE HEALTH CARE INDUSTRY

The history of occupational safety and health regulations in the health care industry is short. The first Occupational Safety and Health Administration (OSHA) standards ever to apply to health care settings include the ethylene oxide, formaldehyde, radiation standards, and the hazard communication standard, which took effect in 1984 and had little overall impact on health care facilities. It was not until the Service Employees International Union (SEIU) and several other health care unions petitioned OSHA for a bloodborne pathogen standard in 1986 that OSHA began to play a major role in regulating the industry.

There was great opposition to OSHA's proposed bloodborne pathogen standard, especially from the American Dental Association. OSHA reported that it received more than 4,000 written comments to the draft standard, far more than any other OSHA regulation to date. The American Dental Association later took OSHA to court, arguing that the standard intruded on the dentists' right to exercise their professional judgment regarding the need for and use of personal protective equipment. OSHA prevailed, and the standard became effective in December 1991.

Hospitals are regulated by the Joint Commission on Accreditation of Healthcare Organizations (JCAHO) and state health departments, agencies that focus on patient care rather than worker health and safety. The JCAHO is a private organization made up of medical industry members including the American Hospital Association (AHA) and the American Medical Association (AMA). The JCAHO has many standards; however, compliance with these standards is voluntary. In contrast, OSHA's mandate is to ensure that employers provide workers with a place of employment free from recognized hazards. Employers who violate OSHA standards are cited and fined.

OSHA's bloodborne pathogen standard reflected not only a growing awareness and concern for the high rate of injury and disease in the health care industry, but it also signaled a major change in focus for OSHA. The fact that 200–300 health care workers die annually because of workplace exposure to the hepatitis B virus received little attention before the advent of the human immunodeficiency virus (HIV).[9] This revelation has led OSHA as well as the JCAHO to pay greater attention to the myriad and widespread injuries and illnesses prevalent in the health care industry.

In 1992, according to the Bureau of Labor Statistics, health care workers had more injuries and illnesses than either miners or construction workers. SEIU and other unions are demanding that greater attention be paid to these problems and that strong regulations designed to prevent exposures to infectious diseases as well as injuries such as back sprains and strains be promulgated expeditiously.

THE FIGHT TO PROTECT HEALTH CARE WORKERS FROM OCCUPATIONAL EXPOSURE TO BLOODBORNE DISEASES: LESSONS LEARNED

In the mid 1980s, SEIU began its campaign to protect health care workers from exposure to infectious disease. Under the banner of "Infection Protection NOW," SEIU's campaign focused on preventing occupational exposure to bloodborne diseases, specifically hepatitis B, hepatitis C, and HIV. SEIU's campaign included developing educational materials and providing training programs to hundreds of SEIU's leaders, rank and file members, and staff on the risks of exposure to bloodborne diseases and methods to control exposures. The union developed a rank and file campaign that included the filing of grievances and bargaining for contract language. Through these methods, the union achieved strong infection control programs on a facility-by-facility basis. However, a national campaign to establish industry-wide standards to protect health care workers from occupational exposure to bloodborne diseases was needed. In 1986, along with several other unions, SEIU petitioned OSHA for a standard to protect workers from occupational exposure to bloodborne diseases. After 6 years and an act of Congress, an OSHA standard was finally promulgated in 1991.

SEIU's effort to achieve standards to protect workers from occupational exposure to bloodborne diseases provided some important lessons that the union is building into its efforts to protect workers from occupational exposure to TB. They are as follows:

1. OSHA must expedite rulemaking on standards to protect health care workers from occupational hazards. During the six years SEIU campaigned for a standard regarding bloodborne pathogens, more than 1,000 workers were estimated to have died from complications associated with contracting hepatitis B on the job. The union believes that the health care industry cannot wait 6 years for OSHA to promulgate a standard to protect workers from TB. To date nationwide, 17 health care workers have developed active multidrug-resistant tuberculosis (MDR-TB); five health care workers have died; and at least several hundred workers have become infected after workplace exposure to TB and have required medical treatment.[6] A survey conducted by the CDC and the AHA found that MDR-TB is widespread in the U.S. and that many hospital TB infection control programs do not meet the CDC's guidelines for preventing occupational transmission of TB. A quarter of the hospitals surveyed reported no rooms meeting CDC criteria for acid-fast bacillus (AFB) isolation. Thirteen percent of the hospitals reported nosocomial TB transmission to health care workers.[7]

In August 1993, SEIU and four other unions petitioned OSHA to initiate rulemaking on a standard to protect workers from occupational exposure to TB. To get OSHA to act expeditiously, SEIU plans to wage a rank and file campaign, as it did on bloodborne diseases, that includes a campaign to keep pressure on the Department of Labor to act swiftly.

2. In the union's opinion, health care workers, management, and government were not seeing the big picture. The union believes that the health care industry must treat every exposure to TB as a significant event. In its effort to protect health care workers, the union has taught its members that every needlestick injury is a significant event that can put a health care worker at risk for infection with hepatitis and HIV. SEIU is currently educating health care workers that the conversion to a positive PPD skin-test represents a significant change in health status. Chemoprophylaxis with isoniazid and other drugs can cause severe side effects. The CDC has recently received reports of severe isoniazid-associated hepatitis. In the case of MDR-TB, drug therapy may be ineffective.

3. Like many other occupational injuries and illnesses, exposure to bloodborne diseases or TB is too often seen as the fault of the worker. SEIU sees this as a dangerous myth. For years, health care workers have been told by management: "If you had only slowed down, thought about what you were doing and been more careful, you would have prevented your injury or exposure." The reality of the health care workplace is short staffing, lack of safety equipment, and lack of worker health and safety training and education.

In SEIU's fight to protect health care workers from occupational exposure to bloodborne diseases, the union pressured management for a commitment to develop strong infection control programs that were based on a hierarchy of controls with engineering controls as the first line of defense. The same is true in its fight for TB standards: SEIU is demanding a TB control program that is based on a hierarchy of controls, including administrative and engineering controls to eliminate or reduce occupational exposure to TB.

4. The union can begin to set standards for controlling exposure to TB through collective bargaining and filing of grievances. Knowing that the fight to get OSHA to promulgate a standard to protect health care workers from bloodborne diseases could take years, the union felt that, in the meantime, it had a tremendous responsibility to begin to set standards for the industry. In the mid 1980s various SEIU local unions began to bargain for strong contract language to protect health care workers from occupational exposure to bloodborne diseases. They won contract language that provided the hepatitis B vaccine free and infection control programs based on universal precautions. In addition, some contracts provided for the formation of joint labor/management needlestick prevention committees to study the rate of needlestick injuries and to research and test safer devices. The right also was won to receive information on a regular basis regarding the number and causes of injuries and illnesses in health care facilities.

Across the country, SEIU local unions are beginning to negotiate contract language that provides for strong TB control programs that are based on a hierarchy of controls and to have access to PPD skin-test conversion data in order to assess the risk of exposure.

5. It is critical to build a record through government agencies, like OSHA, recognizing that exposure to TB is a serious occupational hazard. This can be done through the filing of OSHA complaints under its general duty clause. Before OSHA promulgated its bloodborne disease standard, SEIU local unions were filing complaints with OSHA and getting citations issued against hospitals and other health care facilities under OSHA's general duty clause. Through these citations and subsequent abatement programs, standards were set for the industry regarding how to control bloodborne exposures. In addition, the union began to build a record that demonstrated how facilities throughout the country were not in compliance with CDC's recommended guidelines for protecting health care workers from occupational exposure to bloodborne diseases. This created a record that supported our demands for an OSHA standard that would mandate requirements for employers.

Through the Labor Coalition to Fight TB In the Workplace, several unions petitioned OSHA in December 1992 to release a national compliance guideline providing enforcement guidance on occupational exposure to TB. In response to this petition, OSHA issued a memorandum in August 1993 to provide clarification for OSHA-wide enforcement policy and procedures for inspections concerning occupational exposure to TB. Pending release of the CDC's final revision of its 1990 guidelines for preventing the transmission of TB in health care settings, OSHA will issue a more formal compliance directive.

Prior to the release of OSHA's memorandum, several SEIU local unions had filed complaints with OSHA regarding failure of a hospital to provide adequate protection from exposure to TB. Serious citations were issued at Meriter Hospital in Madison, Wisconsin, Harbor Medical Center in Los Angeles, St. Lukes Hospital in San Francisco, and several correctional facilities.

Under OSHA's enforcement memorandum, SEIU will continue to file complaints wherever we believe the industry is failing to protect workers from exposure to TB.

6. The Centers for Disease Control and Prevention has a critical role to play in protecting health care workers from occupational exposure to infectious diseases. SEIU learned from its experience in protecting health care workers from exposure to bloodborne diseases that the agency had traditionally communicated with the management sector of the health care industry. During the campaign for the bloodborne disease standard, the agency worked with employee representatives and unions for the first time in the health care industry.

Specifically, the Hospital Infections Program of CDC has a great deal of knowledge in the area of infection control, especially in the prevention of nosocomial infections. Moreover, the Hospital Infections Program can become even more effective by working closely with the NIOSH and to generally integrate industrial hygiene principles into the area of infection control.

By providing guidelines to the health care industry that integrate industrial hygiene principles as the main control methods of occupational exposure to TB, the CDC will greatly enhance efforts to protect workers, which is essential during the resurgence of TB.

7. The general public has an obvious interest in being protected from exposure to TB. Education of the public about worker exposure is essential to winning a change in public policy. As part of SEIU's fight to win strong protection for health care workers from occupational exposure to bloodborne diseases, the union stressed that protecting health care workers form unsafe working conditions allowed health care workers to provide good quality and compassionate care to patients.

SEIU wants the public to become well-informed consumers of health care services. The public has a right to be able to evaluate the infection control practices of their health care providers or facilities.

Similarly, SEIU must teach the public that patient-to-patient and patient-to-worker transmission are related and can both be avoided by the use of proper controls to reduce TB exposure.

CASE STUDY: PROTECTING WORKERS FROM EXPOSURE TO TB AT JACKSON MEMORIAL HOSPITAL

On Friday, October 12, 1990, the CDC reported the first cases of nosocomial transmission of multidrug-resistant tuberculosis to health care workers and HIV-infected patients. The incidents occurred at Jackson Memorial Hospital in Miami, the second largest hospital in the U.S. and the sole public hospital for Dade County.

The CDC reported that from January 1988 through July 1990, 10 of the 28 (36%) health care workers on the HIV ward and 3 of the 12 (25%) susceptible health care workers in the HIV clinic had documented skin-test conversions. In addition, the CDC reported that the probable periods of exposure for the 10 health care converters on the HIV ward coincided with the periods that patients who were sputum AFB-smear-positive were hospitalized on that ward.[2]

The CDC investigated the outbreak and asked NIOSH to evaluate the existing control methods in the hospital, including the ventilation system, work practices, and administrative controls on the HIV ward and the HIV clinic. NIOSH reported the following conditions existed on the HIV ward prior to May 1990: Doors of AFB isolation rooms were often left open, and patients were allowed to move freely outside of their rooms, often forgetting to wear their masks. Particulate masks were improperly used by health care workers and visitors. The two patient rooms that were regularly used for respiratory therapy, the administration of pentamidine, and sputum inductions were not provided with proper ventilation; health care workers were simply told to vacate the room during cough-inducing procedures. In addition, health care workers reported minimal contact with the hospital's infection control department regarding TB control methods.[4]

NIOSH learned that in May 1990, the hospital changed policies on the HIV ward that required patient rooms to have a closed door policy, and automatic double entrance doors were installed at both ends of the unit corridor.

In the HIV clinic, NIOSH reported that it was past practice for pentamidine to be administered to several patients in the same area at one time. Patients would receive the treatment and sit in the patient lounge area of the clinic. NIOSH found out that Jackson Memorial Hospital had recently changed the policy to allow only one patient per treatment area and to have the patient remain in the areas for 30 minutes.

SEIU learned of the outbreak prior to the release of the report by CDC when nurses interested in organizing a union at Jackson Memorial Hospital contacted SEIU. In the fall of 1990, SEIU began to build an organizing committee with the nurses at Jackson Memorial Hospital. Fighting for a strong TB control program became a major issue for the nurses' organizing committee and subsequently during the bargaining campaign. During the organizing campaign, nurses began to meet with hospital administrators to voice their concerns about the lack of effective TB control measures. In addition, nurses demanded representation as part of the hospital's efforts to control occupational exposure to TB. The organizing committee requested data on skin-test conversions, reviewed TB policies, and made recommendations for strengthening TB policies. With the assistance of SEIU, the organizing committee sponsored a conference on airborne and bloodborne infectious diseases.

The NIOSH report of January 15, 1991, to Jackson Memorial Hospital included recommendations for controlling the transmission of tuberculosis.[4] NIOSH's first recommendation was to obtain the services of a qualified industrial hygienist to address the wide variety of health and safety hazards found in the hospital. NIOSH recommended that an industrial hygienist should work closely with the hospital's infection control department to prevent transmission of infectious diseases to health care workers.

Several of NIOSH's recommendations addressed the need for further evaluation of the ventilation system in other areas of the hospital, evaluation of exposure to pentamidine, review of the hospital's ultraviolet lamp protocol, and an epidemiologic study of TB conversions. NIOSH stated that follow-up on those recommendations was dependent on a request from the hospital for NIOSH to return to the hospital and conduct further evaluations and studies. However, the hospital failed to invite NIOSH to return to the facility.

The hospital began to implement some of the recommendations from the CDC/NIOSH report. A TB infection control coordinator was hired. Policies were implemented requiring patients on respiratory precautions to stay in their rooms. Booths were installed on the HIV ward and clinic for the administration of pentamidine. Modifications were made in patient rooms to create negative pressure isolation rooms on the HIV ward. High-efficiency particulate air (HEPA) filters were installed, and a more efficient exhaust system was designed. A trailer was approved for use at the TB clinic to handle all patients with suspect or active TB and other respiratory diseases. Plans for the installation and usage of ultraviolet lamps were developed for the general patient areas.

Serious problems still existed. Isolation rooms on the HIV unit and respiratory unit continued to convert back and forth between positive and negative pressure. Workers who administered pentamidine in the newly installed booths continued to have health problems, and skin-test conversions continued to occur. It was clear that the hospital needed to hire a qualified industrial hygienist who could work on site and be involved in the overall plan for controlling TB throughout the facility.

In March 1991, after several more skin-test conversions among health care workers, the organizing committee developed a set of demands to strengthen the TB controls at the hospital. These demands went directly to the Public Health Trust Board, which has oversight for the hospital.

The organizing committee decided to request a health hazard evaluation (HHE) from NIOSH in the spring of 1991, because skin-test conversions continued to occur at Jackson Memorial Hospital. In addition, the nurses were concerned that the hospital was not adequately addressing CDC/NIOSH's recommendations. The organizing committee requested that NIOSH conduct a study of the TB skin-test conversions among the hospital staff. In addition, they requested an evaluation of the newly implemented TB control measures, including the ventilation system in various areas of the hospital, ultraviolet lamp installation and usage, and the hospital's respiratory protection program.

NIOSH returned to the hospital in early May to begin the evaluation. Nurse representatives from the organizing committee participated as walk-around representatives during the course of the entire investigation. NIOSH's presence in the facility acted as an impetus for the hospital to move at a faster pace to implement various control measures. The NIOSH investigation continued into 1992. Throughout NIOSH's investigation, nurses were still concerned that the hospital continued to move slowly over critical issues to protect workers from exposure to TB. While nurses continued to wait for the hospital to implement all of the control measures, seven health care workers were exposed to a single patient with active TB in the operating room.

Angered over the hospital's refusal to respond to the demands for the quick implementation of strong TB control measures, more than 250 nurses filed a class-action grievance demanding action. The grievance focused mainly on the hospital's failure to hire an industrial hygienist, but it also cited the hospital's failure to (1) prohibit a hospital policy that allowed nurses to report their own TB skin-test results; (2) develop a written respiratory program; and (3) provide a timeline for instituting controls and policies to control TB within the county jail system.

In October 1991, the nurses voted overwhelmingly to be represented by SEIU. The union's win at Jackson Memorial Hospital brought SEIU its one millionth member, and SEIU became the fastest growing union within the AFL-CIO.

With the NIOSH investigation continuing and the class-action grievance pending, health and safety continued to be a major issue as nurses began to organize for a strong contract. Comprehensive health and safety language was proposed during contract negotiations. SEIU won precedent-setting contract language that established (1) a comprehensive TB contol program based on industrial hygiene principles, (2) protection from hazards created by new equipment, medical treatment, and/or processes prior to their implementation, such as the administration of aerosolized medications, and (3) the formation of a joint labor/management health and safety committee with broad powers to investigate the workplace and the authority to make recommendations to correct hazardous working conditions.

NIOSH's health hazard evaluation report of November 24, 1992, recommended the use of local exhaust ventilation as the preferred type of ventilation.[5] In addition, NIOSH communicated to Jackson Memorial Hospital in a correspondence dated October 16, 1992, the preliminary results of the study assessing the risk of PPD skin-test conversions among health care workers. The preliminary data revealed that exposed workers had a three times greater risk of conversion than unexposed workers from January 1, 1989, through October 31, 1990. Even after the hospital began to implement control measures, workers continued to convert to TB positive. The skin-test conversion rate actually decreased for the exposed workers beginning in 1991; however, their conversion rate was still significantly higher than for the unexposed workers.[1]

The fight for a strong TB control program continues at Jackson Memorial Hospital. The hospital has finally responded to several issues raised in the class-action grievance. A timeline was developed for implementing TB control measures within the county jail system. A written respirator program was developed, and nurses were provided information on the use of particulate masks. Through the union representatives to the joint labor/management health and safety committee, the union continues to work on resolving two major outstanding issues in the class-action grievance: (1) to end the policy of self-reporting PPD skin-test results and (2) to hire an industrial hygienist.

To summarize, nurses at Jackson Memorial Hospital organized for strong representation on conditions of their work, including protection from unsafe working conditions. Their fight demonstrated that strong protection for health care workers from occupational exposure to TB and other unsafe working conditions can be won through a strong union organization. The formation of a joint labor/management health and safety committee allowed frontline nurses to share with management their expertise about their work, patient care issues, and their need for workplace control methods to protect them from infectious diseases. The union had important information to share with management about effective control measures to protect them from infectious diseases. The union had important information to share with management about effective control measures, the current status of research, and important developments at other facilities.

More importantly, nurses were able to understand the power of unity and to experience that health care workers can win strong workplace protection when they are organized and united.

THE COSH MODEL

In January 1990, the New York Committee for Occupational Safety and Health (NYCOSH) established an infectious disease committee based on its concern that workers, particularly health care workers, needed more information on the widespread problem of infectious disease transmission in the workplace. The task force focused on education initiatives, holding forums on bloodborne disease prevention and emphasizing the use of engineering controls such as safer medical devices to reduce needlestick injuries.

By 1991, several TB outbreaks had been reported in New York City hospitals and in a prison in upstate New York, which led the committee to change its focus to TB prevention. The committee began to sponsor forums on TB control programs, culminating with a conference entitled *Controlling TB in the Workplace*, which drew 300 participants on October 17, 1993.

The committee plays a vital role in providing updated information on TB controls and recommendations. Many union rank and file workers attend the monthly meetings as well as infection control practitioners, doctors, nurses, orderlies, lab technicians, and nursing home and other health care workers. The committee brings together various members of the hospital hierarchy and facilitates discussion and debate on effective control measures. As a result, educational materials have been developed by and for the committee that review the current federal, state, and city guidelines as well as the OSHA and the New York State Public Employee Safety and Health Bureau (PESH) requirements. Manufacturers were brought in to demonstrate state-of-the-art technology for the control of TB. A survey was also developed to assist rank and file workers and others in evaluating their own workplaces.

One member, a nurse employed at a health care facility in New York, sought the committee's assistance in filing a complaint to OSHA on the facility's lack of a TB control program. When management continued to ignore workers' pleas for a comprehensive TB control plan, she came to committee meetings to educate herself and her coworkers about recommended controls and personal protective equipment. After repeated requests to get management to buy appropriate respirators, health care workers attracted the attention of a New York newspaper when they went out and purchased their own respirators to wear to work each day.

Many members of the NYCOSH infectious disease committee have been active on their facility labor/management committee, and some have filed complaints to OSHA on tuberculosis and other infectious diseases. The committee has provided crucial support to these members in terms of education, training, and strategies for improving TB control plans.

In 1994, the committee cosponsored a forum with OSHA to review the new national OSHA Enforcement Procedures for Tuberculosis. More than 350 workers, union activists, and health care professionals attended the standing-room-only conference. Union activists strongly voiced their belief that TB infection in workers due to occupational exposure is unacceptable. Many articulated the concern that until it can be demonstrated that engineering controls alone provide adequate protection against TB, the use of effective and reliable personal respiratory protection is essential. Finally, workers and labor unions acknowledged that the struggle to win strong comprehensive protection against TB and, ultimately, an OSHA TB standard had just begun.

ROLE OF THE REGULATORY AGENCIES

In the fall of 1991, labor unions representing public employees, health care workers, teachers, and correction workers asked PESH and OSHA to meet and discuss steps that could be taken immediately to protect workers from exposure to tuberculosis. By this time, several documented outbreaks of MDR-TB had occurred in New York. Unions argued that there was sufficient cause to use OSHA's general duty clause, which states that "employers have a general duty to provide a workplace which is free from recognized hazards." Since TB has long been recognized as a hazard, SEIU strongly urged PESH and OSHA to apply this important provision. On November 15, 1991, a worker died after contracting MDR-TB while guarding inmates who were infected with MDR-TB in an upstate New York prison.

PESH released its *Enforcement Guidelines for Occupational Exposure to Tuberculosis* in April 1992, and OSHA Region II followed a month later with guidelines that were almost identical. The only difference between the two was that PESH recommended the use of particulate respirators whereas OSHA *required* them when entering isolation rooms, performing high risk procedures, or transporting patients. Based on the 1990 CDC guidelines, both agencies required free medical screening during work time, respiratory isolation rooms under negative pressure and exhausted to the outside or through HEPA filters, and warning signs listing precautions posted on the door.

These enforcement procedures addressed only public employers in New York state and private employers in OSHA's Region II, which includes New York, New Jersey, and Puerto Rico. Because PESH and OSHA were using the general duty clause and not a specific standard, they relied on the CDC recommendations, which identified the following high-risk populations: (1) health care settings, (2) correctional institutions, (3) homeless shelters, (4) long-term care facilities, and (5) drug treatment centers.

Despite its limited scope, the PESH and OSHA enforcement policy enabled SEIU and other unions to demand minimum protection as outlined in these documents across the country. OSHA began responding to TB complaints from not just New York state but Connecticut, Illinois, and California. SEIU members raised the enforcement policy at joint labor management health and safety committees and introduced contract language during negotiations to secure similar protection.

On October 8, 1993, OSHA issued a national enforcement policy for occupational exposure to TB. In addition to the requirements found in OSHA's Region II policy, two other critical components were included. SEIU argued vigorously that a protocol for early identification and isolation as well as training and information to ensure worker knowledge of TB transmission and controls was essential. OSHA concurred and this is reflected in the national policy.[6]

THE 1990 CDC GUIDELINES

Although many representatives from the health care industry stated that the 1990 CDC guidelines needed implementation but not revision, labor unions voiced strong concern about the guidelines and advised the CDC to revise them extensively. Unions urged the agency to provide a framework for a hierarchy of controls that includes administrative controls, engineering controls, personal protective equipment, and training and education.

Among the major issues raised by unions for CDC consideration were:

- There is no acceptable PPD conversion rate
- The need for a risk assessment that looks at exposures as well as conversions and an assessment of existing engineering controls
- High quality, interactive training for health care workers on TB in a language that workers understand
- The provision of confidential counseling to immunocompromised health care workers with respect to reasonable accommodations and work reassignments
- The use of HEPA filtered respirators as the minimal level of respiratory protection
- Compliance with OSHA's respiratory protection standard.

CDC incorporated many of the comments submitted by SEIU, other unions, and other organizations representing health care workers. When CDC released its draft on August 4, 1993, the document had changed dramatically. The draft guidelines, if finalized without significant changes, will represent a precedent in merging infection control and industrial hygiene principles. It can and will serve as a model for controlling hazards in the health care field.

ORGANIZING TO PROTECT HEALTH CARE WORKERS FROM OCCUPATIONAL EXPOSURE TO TB

Organized labor has already experienced several victories in its fight to protect health care workers from exposure to TB. The CDC listened to the unions' concerns and incorporated into its draft guidelines a hierarchy of controls and good industrial hygiene practices to eliminate or reduce the risk of occupational exposure to TB at its source. OSHA has issued a memorandum that provides guidance on enforcement procedures to OSHA inspectors on occupational exposure to TB. The memorandum covers the application of OSHA standards for TB inspections as well as the OSHA act's general duty clause that obligates employers to provide safe and healthful workplaces. OSHA informed the unions in January 1994 that they agree with the unions' petition for a TB standard and will begin the formal rulemaking process.

These are important steps toward the development of strong standards to protect workers from occupational exposure to TB. SEIU's fight to protect workers from occupational exposure from bloodborne diseases taught the union that it needs to have strong enforcement action to protect workers from hazardous working conditions. OSHA must act quickly to begin rulemaking procedures on a TB standard that clarifies what employers are obligated to do and facilitates enforcement on TB. OSHA has stated that a draft TB rule is expected to be published in the *Federal Register* by April 1995. The CDC's revision to its 1990 guidelines is another important step.

Unions have had a major impact in protecting workers from hazardous working conditions. The Service Employees International Union has been leading the fight to protect health care workers from infectious diseases on both a rank and file and a national level. On a rank and file level SEIU advocates using the grievance procedure, fighting for strong contract language, and using health and safety committees to address unsafe working conditions and file OSHA complaints. On a national level, SEIU will continue to push for enforceable standards that will protect workers from exposure to TB.

REFERENCES

1. Boudreau Y: NIOSH correspondence to Joan Otten, Jackson Memorial Hospital. Cincinnati, NIOSH publication HETA 91-187, October 16, 1992.
2. Centers for Disease Control: Nosocomial transmission of multidrug resistant tuberculosis to health care workers and HIV infected patients in an urban hospital—Florida. MMWR 39:718–722, 1990.
3. Centers for Disease Control: NIOSH recommended guidelines for personal respiratory protection of workers in health-care facilities potentially exposed to tuberculosis. US Dept of Health and Human Services, Atlanta, September 14, 1992.
4. Elliott L, Hughes R, Mortimer V: NIOSH correspondence to Marlene Rifkin, Jackson Memorial Hospital. Cincinnati, NIOSH publication HETA 90-350, January 15, 1991.
5. Klein M, Mortimer V, Decker J, Clark N: NIOSH Health Hazard Evaluation Ventilation Report, Jackson Memorial Hospital. Cincinnati, NIOSH publication HETA 91-187, November 24, 1992.
6. Occupational Safety and Health Administration: Enforcement policy and procedures for occupational exposure to tuberculosis. Washington, DC, October 8, 1993.
7. Rudnick J, Kroc K, Manangan S, et al: How prepared are hospitals to control nosocomial transmission of tuberculosis. Presented at the third annual meeting of the Society for Hospital Epidemiology of America, Chicago, April 18–20, 1993.
8. US Bureau of Labor Statistics: Workplace Injuries and Illnesses in 1992 [press release]. Washington, DC, US Dept of Labor publication, December 15, 1993.
9. US Department of Labor: OSHA Final Rule on Occupational Exposure to Bloodborne Pathogens. Federal Register 56:64003-64182, December 6, 1991.

MELISSA A. McDIARMID, MD, MPH
N.A. GILLEN, BS
LEE HATHON, PE, MSPH

REGULATORY CONSIDERATIONS OF OCCUPATIONAL TUBERCULOSIS CONTROL

From the Occupational Safety and Health Administration
U.S. Department of Labor
Washington, DC

Reprint requests to:
Melissa A. McDiarmid, MD, MPH
U.S. Department of Labor/OSHA
200 Constitution Ave., NW
Room N 3506
Washington, DC 20210

The views presented herein are those of the authors and do not necessarily represent the views of the Occupational Safety and Health Administration.

Tuberculosis has long been recognized as an occupational hazard, with reports of the disease among health care workers dating to the last century.[17] Nonoccupational prevalence of disease has always been a significant factor determining exposure among health care workers. In the 1930s, prior to advances in infection control and chemotherapy, a study of student nurses at Philadelphia General Hospital revealed positive tuberculosis skin tests for 28% of entering students, but 100% for graduates three years later.[6] The 28% rate was presumed to be the background rate in the general population. Clearly, the opportunity for exposure was a reflection of the higher background prevalence and the lack of now recognized infection control techniques.

Classic public health and infection control measures, including early identification and isolation of patients, together with advances in antituberculosis chemotherapy in the middle part of this century, have dramatically lowered the incidence of tuberculosis. These measures prevented disease not only in the general population but also in health care workers so well that, prior to the 1980s, hospital infection control authorities considered TB to be in check in their institutions if annual skin-test conversion rates among workers were about 1–3%.[1,2,23]

In the mid 1980s, however, the declining rate of TB the nation had enjoyed for several decades came to a halt, and rates began to increase. The increase can be attributed to the classic risk factors for TB, includng poverty, overcrowding, homelessness, limited access to health care, poor nutritional status, and other recognized indicators of decline in the nation's social fabric.[18] Long recognized as a disease of poverty, TB continues to be so. The new epidemic is focused on, although not confined to, large urban centers where people with the above risk factors tend to congregate.

An important new factor in the current outbreak, however, is the increase in immunocompromised people exposed to TB. TB is an opportunistic infection in immunocompromised people, including those with HIV infection.[3,19,22] The convergence of immunocompromised people and those who possess the risk factors for TB occurs in both prisons and hosptials. For example, the incidence of HIV infection in prison inmates in New York state increased dramatically from 1976 to 1986, from 15.4 per 100,000 to 105.5 per 100,000.[5] Highly publicized nosocomial TB outbreaks have in several cases been attributed to infection transmitted between hospitals and prisons while care was being rendered to ill inmates.[10]

The Centers for Disease Control and Prevention (CDC) in cooperation with the American Hospital Association (AHA) recently completed a survey of 729 medical institutions. They reported that active TB had occurred in health care workers at 90 (13.1%) of the responding institutions.[24] More than 80% of the responding facilities reported skin-test conversions in health care workers but not active disease. Comprehensive data on work-related TB, even in a health care setting, have been difficult to acquire. One recent review, based on annual screenings of health care workers, documented that skin-test conversion rates ranged from less than 1% to 5% in the 1960s through 1990.[4] Post-exposure conversion rates, however, have been documented in the literature with much higher rates: from 6–77% of health care workers exposed.[4] A significant barrier to obtaining occupational data regarding TB is that, until recently, the form used to report TB cases to the CDC did not collect occupational data. This caused lack of recognition of the disease's relation to work exposures. Clearly, there is a significant work-related component to this epidemic that must be addressed by the regulatory community.

OSHA

The Occupational Safety and Health Act of 1970 provided for the development, promulgation, and enforcement of standards to protect the safety and health of workers. When a serious hazard arises and in the absence of specific standards, the Occupational Safety and Health Administration (OSHA) uses the act's general duty clause (section 5.(a)(1)) to protect workers. The clause states: "Each employer shall furnish to each of his employees employment and a place of employment which are free from recognized hazards that are causing or are likely to cause death or serious physical harm to his employees."[20] OSHA may thus use recognized safety and health standards of practice recommended by consensus standard-setting bodies. These standards, as published in the medical or professional literature, can be seen as methods of abatement in citing exposure of employees to a recognized, serious hazard for which there is a feasible and useful method of control.

In the case of tuberculosis, the CDC is a recognized authority in the health care industry. Specific guidance for controlling TB has been published by the CDC in its *Morbidity and Mortality Weekly Reports* (MMWR) for five high-risk employment settings: health care institutions,[9] correctional facilities,[7] homeless shelters,[12] long-term care for the elderly,[11] and drug treatment centers.[8] Some elements are the same for each setting, such as the early identification and isolation

TABLE 1. Hierarchy of Industrial Hygiene Controls

Substitution
Engineering controls
Negative pressure respiratory isolation
Treatment booth/local exhaust ventilation
Administrative controls
Identification and isolation of patients
Skin test surveillance
Respiratory isolation signs
Controlling traffic in/out of respiratory isolation room
High-hazard procedure practices
Worker training and education
Personal protective equipment
Particulate respirators

of infectious patients, but some unique aspects of the various employment settings require special considerations. This chapter will focus on health care institutions because they allow opportunity for exposure to the greatest number of workers and most worker complaints related to TB investigated by OSHA arise there.

Hierarchy of Industrial Hygiene Controls—Controlling the Hazard

The regulatory approach to occupational TB control derives from the classic hierarchy of workplace controls displayed in Table 1.[25] With TB, however, substitution of a less hazardous substance is not applicable. Preventing TB exposure requires using a combination of controls. Engineering controls, discussed below, play a major role by isolating the hazard from the worker. Administrative and work practice controls reduce time spent with patients and, therefore, exposure to the hazard. In addition to engineering and administrative controls, personal protective equipment (PPE), notably respirators for TB exposure, also will be necessary in some limited areas.

OSHA traditionally allows the use of PPE when engineering, administrative, and work practice controls are not sufficient to protect the worker. OSHA derived the elements for TB exposure control for health care workers from the CDC document addressing the hospital work setting,[9] the elements of which are listed in Table 2.

In the fall of 1993, OSHA issued direction to its compliance officers regarding the conduct of a TB inspection. Titled *Enforcement Policy and Procedures for Occupational Exposure to Tuberculosis*, this document describes elements a high-risk facility must address in controlling occupational exposure to TB[21] (Table 2). As with any other hazard for which there is no specific standard, OSHA first enforces

TABLE 2. Elements of a Tuberculosis Control Plan for Health Care Workers

Written exposure control plan[a]
Identification and isolation of patients
Respiratory isolation rooms
Employee TB surveillance
Respiratory protection
Education and training[b]

[a] = Absence of a written program is not currently cited.
[b] = This element was not included in the CDC's original guidelines but is expected to be included in the update.[14]

its existing standards to protect workers. If these are inadequate for a known hazard, which can be controlled in a recognized manner, Section 5.(a)(1) will be in coverage. This general duty clause can require a variety of controls.

TB Exposure Control Program

Based on CDC recommendations, OSHA requires through its general duty clause that high-hazard facilities develop comprehensive TB exposure control programs that implement a multifaceted approach to controlling occupational TB exposure. They need not be stand-alone programs but may be incorporated into a facility's existing infection control plan.

Since tuberculosis is usually transmitted via the airborne route, prevention can be achieved by minimizing dispersal of the exhaled air of the infected individual. This can be done by preventing the generation of infectious droplet nuclei by early identification and treatment, preventing their spread by controlling the source, reducing microbial contamination of air, and conducting surveillance for tuberculosis transmission to health care facility personnel to minimize further transmission.[9]

Identification and Isolation of Patients

Early identification, isolation, and treatment of people with active disease will reduce the generation of infectious droplets.[9] OSHA expects high-hazard facilities to have an effective program to identify and treat individuals with TB. When possible, a screening procedure should be in place in these facilities. Workers must be trained to have a high index of suspicion for tuberculosis when a patient/client/inmate presents with symptoms consistent with the disease. The facility must have a protocol for isolating and treating such individuals. If this cannot be done on site, there must be a procedure or arrangement to transfer TB patients to facilities capable of doing so.

Respiratory Isolation

Engineering controls function primarily by isolating the hazard from the worker. The use of negative-pressure respiratory isolation rooms for any suspected or known TB patient is an engineering control that will minimize the spread of droplet nuclei outside the patient's room.[9]

Protecting health care workers outside of acid-fast bacillus (AFB) isolation/treatment rooms is achieved by containing TB droplet nuclei within AFB isolation/treatment rooms by using the following engineering and work practice control measures:

- Isolation/treatment rooms in use by patients with suspected and confirmed infectious TB should be kept under sufficient negative pressure to induce airflow into the room from all surrounding spaces, such as the corridor, ceiling plenums, and plumbing chases. Many case studies demonstrate that the loss of containment, or negative pressure, contributes to the risk of infection.[15,17]
- Direction of airflow into isolation/treatment rooms must be demonstrated regularly while the room is being used by patients with suspected and confirmed infectious TB. The employer should demonstrate that direction of airflow is from the corridor into the isolation/treatment room with the door closed, using smoke trails or some other indicator at the door transfer grille or undercut. If an anteroom exists, demonstration of direction of airflow should occur at the inner door between the isolation/treatment room and the anteroom.

- Air from isolation/treatment rooms should be exhausted directly to the outside in ducts labeled as transporting contagious air. In addition, these contagious air ducts must be kept under negative pressure until the exhaust air is discharged outside safely (away from occupied areas and air intakes) or decontaminated by a recognized process (such as high-efficiency filtration). The intent is to prevent cross-contamination between the exhaust air from isolation/treatment rooms and the rest of the health care setting. Ducts and fans that transport TB contagious air must be labeled in order to protect maintenance personnel.
- Opening and closing of doors in an isolation/treatment room that does not have an anteroom compromises the ability to maintain negative pressure in the room. For these rooms, the employer must use a combination of controls and practices to minimize spillage of contaminated air into the corridor. Recognized controls and practices include but are not limited to minimizing entry to room, adjusting the hydraulic closer so that doors open and close slowly to reduce displacement effects, having doors swing into the room in the direction of airflow when fire codes permit, avoiding locating room exhaust intake near doors, and using phones to communicate with the patient.

In order to protect health care workers *inside* AFB isolation/treatment rooms, engineering controls should be used to kill, remove, and/or dilute TB droplet nuclei to the lowest feasible level. Ventilation with uncontaminated air will sweep and dilute TB droplet nuclei from the room. The American Society of Heating, Refrigerating and Air-Conditioning Engineers recommends a ventilation rate of six air changes per hour (ACH) for isolation rooms for the comfort of the patient. At this ventilation rate and assuming perfect mixing in the room *and no further generation of the contaminant*, it would take 46 minutes to theoretically remove 99% of the airborne contaminants. The CDC recognizes germicidal ultraviolet irradiation as a supplement to general ventilation to kill TB bacilli in the isolation/treatment room. Stand-alone, portable, high-efficiency particulate air (HEPA) filtration units operating within isolation/treatment rooms could also augment general ventilation by further removing TB bacilli from the air by recirculating room air through a HEPA filter. It may be difficult to support a specific recommended minimum general ventilation rate due to lack of definitive data from well-designed, direct studies regarding the efficacy of general ventilation in reducing risk of exposure to TB. However, it is recommended and encouraged that general ventilation rates exceeding minimums be considered.

Once the engineering controls are in place, they can be enhanced by the use of such administrative and work practice controls as performing high-hazard procedures in the negative pressure isolation rooms. A high-hazard procedure is one that has the potential to generate airborne respiratory secretions; examples are sputum induction, aerosolized medication administration, bronchoscopy, endotracheal suctioning, and some autopsy procedures. When the procedure cannot be done in the patient's room, it should take place in a negative-pressure treatment room. When possible, local exhaust ventilation for the specific procedure should be used.

Employee traffic into the isolation areas should be minimized by combining as many tasks as possible into one visit. When feasible, and if appropriate, employees may interview the patient/client by telephone, which will reduce the time of employee exposure in the isolation area. Consistent with good medical practice, elective procedures should be delayed until the patient is noninfectious.

Local Source Capture Ventilation

Due to the inefficiency of general ventilation, much more emphasis must be placed on engineering control solutions that prevent or contain TB droplet nuclei at their source. When feasible without compromising medical procedures, local source capture ventilation should be used to entrap infectious droplets whenever cough-inducing or aerosol-generating high-risk procedures are performed. Local source control ventilation devices include full containment enclosures such as booths and tents and partial enclosures such as hoods or snorkels.

Laboratories

Aerosol-generating manipulations of clinical specimens of *Mycobacterium tuberculosis* in mycobacteriology laboratories must be conducted in class I or II biological safety cabinets (BSC). Biological safety cabinets must be recertified annually at a minimum, when the HEPA filters are changed, and when the BSC is moved or undergoes maintenance.[13]

Some procedures involving *Mycobacterium tuberculosis* in mycobacteriology laboratories mandate Biosafety Level 3 facilities, which require that the laboratory be under negative pressure compared to surrounding spaces and be accessed only through an anteroom. Per the advisory guidelines in the CDC/NIH publication, *Biosafety in Microbiological and Biomedical Laboratories*, the laboratory director is responsible for recommending the appropriate biosafety level after assessing risks of the activities involved.

Employee TB Surveillance Program

A medical surveillance program for the high-risk facilities must be established to identify personnel with tuberculous infection without evidence of active disease. Preventive treatment may be indicated for these individuals, and this type of medical surveillance will also allow the facility to evaluate the effectiveness of its exposure control program.[9]

OSHA expects facilities to follow the current CDC recommendations for medical surveillance. The purpose and interpretation of TB skin testing, including the significance of a skin-test conversion, must be explained to employees so that they may make an informed decision about participating in the program. It has never been OSHA's policy to force employees to accept medical treatment or testing. It is, however, the employer's responsibility to make medical surveillance and treatment available at a reasonable time and place and at no cost to the employee.

As discussed above, although OSHA has no specific TB standard, some of its existing standards can be applied to worker protection against tuberculosis. Records of skin testing results, medical evaluations, chest x-ray results, and treatments are considered employee medical records that in accordance with 29 CFR 1910.20 must be preserved and maintained for at least the duration of employment plus 30 years.

Recording Occupational Illnesses

29 CFR 1904 covers the recording and reporting of occupational injuries and illnesses. Tuberculosis infections (positive skin test) and tuberculosis disease are both recordable on the OSHA 200 log in facilities where tuberculosis has been identified as a hazard, such as correctional facilities and drug treatment centers. A positive skin test for tuberculosis, even on baseline testing (except pre-employment

screening), is recordable on the OSHA 200 log because there is a presumption of work-relatedness in these facilities. However, if an employee is found to have a positive skin test but was also positive prior to employment, the case would not be recordable.

If an employee's tuberculosis infection progresses to disease during employment, the case would also be recordable on the OSHA 200 log because of the presumption of work-related exposure in these settings and because the findings represent an abnormal condition or disorder caused by exposure to environmental factors associated with employment that may be caused by inhalation [Recordkeeping Guideline for Occupational Injuries and Illnesses, 29 CFR 1904]. This information would be important to employers who are evaluating the efficacy of their tuberculosis control program.

If an employer has never provided testing to employees, an unusually high number of cases can be expected to be recorded the first year of recordkeeping. This should not cause undue alarm. The OSHA 200 log does not determine eligibility for workers' compensation cases and does not automatically trigger an OSHA inspection. The goal of recordkeeping is to provide accurate data to aid the employer in designing an effective program. If unusually high TB rates are identified through recordkeeping, the next step is to evaluate the tuberculosis control program to determine its effectiveness.

When baseline and periodic skin test results are performed and recorded correctly, tuberculosis infection and incidence rates in workers can and should be calculated. This will enable employers to identify the risk of tuberculosis transmission to various work groups, evaluate the effectiveness of the exposure-control practices at the worksite, and make appropriate policy to afford employee protection.

As with all medical records, TB-related medical records must be maintained confidentially and in accordance with federal, state, and local regulations.

Labeling Requirements

The use of a biohazard label is required by 29 CFR 1910.145. The infectious patient/client should be easily identifiable by employees so that proper precautions can be taken. Labels on the isolation area door and indicators printed on the client's record in easily recognized language or symbols are methods to meet this requirement. The indicators should continue to be used if the infectious patient is moved to another location. During recent OSHA inspections, a common preprinted "Respiratory Isolation" sign was found to use unacceptable wording. It states: "Masks are indicated for those who come *close* to patient." Respiratory protection must be donned before entering the room.

Worker Training

Providing training to ensure employee knowledge of TB hazards, including transmission, signs and symptoms, medical surveillance, therapy, and site-specific protocols, is necessary to control the occupational transmission of TB. Such training enhances employees' ability to identify and recognize active TB in patients, coworkers, and themselves and reinforces the need to comply with site-specific control methods and safe work practices.

Respiratory Protection

29 CFR 1910.134(a)(2) requires the provision of respirators that are "applicable and suitable for the purpose intended." Since TB is transmitted solely by

inhalation of airborne droplet nuclei contaminated with *Mycobacterium tuberculosis*, good industrial hygiene practice would dictate the use of respirators in certain high hazard situations. OSHA requires that employees must be provided with and wear NIOSH-certified HEPA respirators or respirators affording greater protection, under the following circumstances:

- When entering a pulmonary isolation room occupied by a patient with known or suspected infectious tuberculosis
- While performing certain high-hazard medical procedures, such as aerosol administration of medication (pentamidine), bronchoscopy, and diagnostic sputum induction. Such procedures pose a much higher risk of aerosolization of *Mycobacterium tuberculosis* and, thus, transmission of TB to others.
- When transporting TB patients

All of the above exposures involve direct employee contact with patients known or strongly suspected to be infectious. While other elements of the TB employee protection program must address the protection of employees with repeated, prolonged contact with high-risk patients, whose TB status is not known, OSHA does not require the use of respiratory protection by those employees at present. Until NIOSH determines an appropriate respirator for TB, OSHA will accept HEPA or any more effective respiratory protection.

OSHA expects its compliance safety and health officers to avoid exposure to any potentially infectious situations when they can be reasonably anticipated. However, if the health officers feel it is necessary to enter isolation areas for compliance purposes, they will wear appropriate respiratory protection. The employer shall institute a respiratory protection program in accordance with the respirator standard 1910.134.

CONCLUSION

The resurgence of tuberculosis, complicated by multidrug-resistant strains, is a significant challenge to the regulatory community's responsibility to ensure the health of exposed workers. The classic hierarchy of industrial hygiene controls may, however, be successfully used to control the hazard. Another element that is critical for effective tuberculosis control is resurrecting the public health infrastructure of early identification, isolation, and treatment of patients, an approach that was once enormously effective in managing this disease. These traditional approaches remain viable methods of reducing the present-day hazard of occupational tuberculosis.

REFERENCES

1. American Hospital Association: Guidelines on Tuberculosis Control Programs for Hospital Employees 49:57–60, 1975.
2. Atuk NO, Hunt EH: Serial tuberculosis testing and isoniazid therapy in general hospital employees. JAMA 218:1795–1798, 1971.
3. Barnes PF, Bloch AB, Davidson PT, Snider DE Jr: Current concepts: Tuberculosis in patients with human immunodeficiency virus infection. N Engl J Med 324:1644–1650, 1991.
4. Bowden K, McDiarmid MA: Occupationally acquired tuberculosis: What's known. J Occup Med 36:302–325, 1994.
5. Braun MM, Truman BI, Maguire B, et al: Increasing incidence of tuberculosis in a prison inmate population. JAMA 261:393–397, 1989.
6. Catanzaro A: Nosocomial tuberculosis. Am Rev Respir Dis 125:559–562, 1982.
7. Centers for Disease Control: Control of tuberculosis in correctional facilitites: A guide for health care workers. Atlanta, Centers for Disease Control, 1991.
8. Centers for Disease Control: Transmission of MDR-TB from an HIV-positive client in a residential substance-abuse treatment facility—Michigan. MMWR 40(RR-8):129–131, 1991.

9. Centers for Disease Control: Guidelines for preventing the transmission of tuberculosis in health care settings, with special focus on HIV-related issues. MMWR 39(RR-17):1–29, 1990.
10. Centers for Disease Control: Nosocomial transmission of multidrug-resistant tuberculosis among HIV-infected persons—Florida and New York, 1988–1991. MMWR 40:585–591, 1991.
11. Centers for Disease Control: Prevention and control of tuberculosis in facilities providing long-term care to the elderly. MMWR 39(RR-10):7–10, 1990.
12. Centers for Disease Control: Tuberculosis control among homeless populations. MMWR 36:May 8, 1987.
13. Centers for Disease Control: Biosafety in Microbiological and Biomedical Laboratories. 3rd ed. Atlanta, Centers for Disease Control, 1993.
14. Centers for Disease Control and Prevention: Draft guidelines for preventing the transmission of tuberculosis in health care facilities, 2nd ed; Notice of comment period. Federal Register 58:52810–52854, October 12, 1993.
15. Edlin BR, Tokars JI, Grieco MH, et al: An outbreak of multi-drug resistant tuberculosis among hospitalized patients with the acquired immunodeficiency syndrome. N Engl J Med 326:1514–1521, 1992.
16. Geiseler PJ, Nelson KE, Crispen RG, Moses VK: Tuberculosis in physicians: A continuing problem. Am Rev Respir Dis 133:773–778, 1986.
17. Hutton M, Stead W, Cauthen G, et al: Nosocomial transmission of tuberculosis associated with a draining abscess. J Infect Dis 161:286–295, 1990.
18. Joseph S: Tuberculosis, again [editorial]. Am J Public Health 83:647–648, 1993.
19. Nolan CM: Human immunodeficiency syndrome-associated tuberculosis: A review with an emphasis on infection control issues. Am J Infect Control 20:30–34, 1992.
20. Occupational Safety and Health Act, Public Law 91-596, Department of Labor, Washington, DC, 1970.
21. Occupational Safety and Health Administration: Enforcement Policy and Procedures for Occupational Exposures to Tuberculosis. Washington, DC, October 8, 1993.
22. Pitchenik AE, Burr J, Suarez M, et al: Human T-cell lymphotrophic virus-III (HTLV-III) seropositivity and related diseases among 71 consecutive patients in whom tuberculosis was diagnosed: A prospective study. Am Rev Respir Dis 135:875–879, 1987.
23. Riley RA: The hazard is relative. Am Rev Respir Dis 96:623–625, 1967.
24. Rudnick J, Krock K, Manangan L, et al: How prepared are U.S. hospitals to control nosocomial transmission of tuberculosis? [abstract]. Presented at the Society of Hospital Epidemiologists of America. Chicago, April 1993.
25. Soule RD: Industrial hygiene engineering controls. In Clayton GD, Clayton FE (eds): Patty's Industrial Hygiene and Toxicoloy. 3rd ed. New York, John Wiley & Sons, 1978.

LISA H. WATSON, MPH
JONATHAN D. ROSEN, BS

EDUCATING WORKERS ABOUT TUBERCULOSIS

From the New York Committee for Occupational Safety and Health
New York, New York (LHW)
and
Department of Occupational Health and Safety
New York State Public Employees Federation
AFL-CIO
Albany, New York (JDR)

Reprint requests to:
Lisa H. Watson
New York Committee for Occupational Safety and Health
275 Seventh Avenue
New York, NY 10001

At a state penitentiary, workers are told that the communicable disease unit is a safe environment in which to work due to the negative air pressure in the isolation rooms and the improved ventilation system. However, nobody is trained to monitor the system or understands the role of negative air pressure, and isolation room doors are occasionally left open. As a result, workers are reluctant to work in the unit.

At a soup kitchen, workers refuse to serve people with HIV due to fear of tuberculosis transmission. They have heard that people infected with HIV are likely to have TB and, therefore, to protect themselves, they feel the soup kitchen should not serve people with HIV.

In a large, urban social service agency, workers buy masks and begin wearing them to work when they hear a coworker has tuberculosis. Pictures of them in the newspaper instigate a string of similar actions in other agencies.

Emergency room workers in a city hospital have been told they are not at increased risk of contracting TB, because they do not have prolonged contact with infectious patients. However, when they discover that several coworkers tested positive on PPD screening tests, they go to their union demanding action.

Tuberculosis presents a formidable challenge for workplace safety and health. While federal, state, and city agencies debate the efficacy of protective measures such as respirators and ultraviolet lights, workers need to learn as much as possible about the disease in order to play an active role in assessing their own risk, ensuring that necessary protections are in place, monitoring the workplace, and contributing to a TB control program. Early identification and isolation of people suspected or known to have TB are essential aspects of controlling exposure on the job, but only worker education can provide the link between policy and implementation.

Very few models of workplace TB training curricula exist. The dearth of educational programs is a direct result of the decreased funding for TB control that occurred in the early 1980s. Most institutions simply do not teach workers about this disease. The majority of existing educational programs tend to focus narrowly on its medical aspects while omitting other key information on environmental controls, workplace practices, and the social context of its resurgence.

Reports of TB transmission within various work settings in the past 2–3 years reinforce the urgent need for the development of workpalce TB prevention programs with a strong educational component.

- The Centers for Disease Control investigated nine outbreaks of multidrug-resistant TB from 1990 through 1992 in a variety of institutional settings. At least 17 workers developed active MDR-TB as a result of these outbreaks.[19]
- A recently published study of a New York City hospital documented a 22–50% skin-test conversion rate among health care workers assigned to wards where TB patients were hospitalized.[17,18]
- In October 1991, a New York state correction officer died of MDR-TB after contracting it from an inmate.[13,14] At the time, he was providing security for sick inmates at an upstate medical center. During March–November 1991, 18 inmates in New York state correctional facilities died from MDR-TB.[14]

In response to the rise in multidrug-resistant tuberculosis in New York City over the past few years, the New York Committee for Occupational Safety and Health (NYCOSH) and the Hunter College Center on AIDS, Drugs and Community Health have developed and conducted training programs on TB for a variety of affected workers, employers, and clients. This chapter is based on the experience of Hunter's AIDS center, NYCOSH, and the New York State Public Employees Federation (PEF), one of NYCOSH's member unions, in developing TB education programs.

EDUCATION: A KEY COMPONENT OF A WORKPLACE TB PREVENTION PROGRAM

The goal of a workplace TB control program is to reduce occupational exposure to prevent workers from developing TB infection and disease. Effective programs will increase the capacity of workers to assess workplace hazards and to take action to reduce these hazards. Thus, knowledge-building is essential for successful implementation of any TB prevention program.

TB education should both inform and motivate. With knowledge and a sense of purpose, workers can respond to situations that put them at risk of exposure. Furthermore, trained workers can assist in determining the needs of the workplace, develop and monitor a workplace TB prevention program, and pass information on to coworkers and clients.

The Centers for Disease Control's draft *Guidelines for Preventing the Transmission of Tuberculosis in Health Care Facilities*[12] highlight the need for "early detection, isolation and treatment of persons with active TB" as the cornerstone of a prevention program. However, poverty, ignorance, and lack of access to health care inhibit many people in affected populations from receiving adequate treatment and care, perpetuating a cycle of contagion, morbidity, and mortality. Clearly, educated workers who serve populations at risk of developing disease can play a vital role in ensuring that patients with infectious TB are quickly identified, appropriately isolated, and properly treated.

The CDC's 1993 draft guidelines, which are expected to be finalized in late 1994, emphasize the importance of the following elements of a TB prevention program: "(1) the hierarchy of control measures including administrative and engineering controls, and personal respiratory protection, (2) health-care facility risk assessment and development of a written TB control plan, (3) early detection and management of persons with TB, (4) purified protein derivative (PPD) skin testing programs, and (5) health-care worker (HCW) education."[2] Clearly, a comprehensive education program is the key link between TB policy and implementation.

WORKER INVOLVEMENT IN TB EDUCATION PROGRAMS

Worker involvement should be integrated into every element of a TB worksite prevention program. Who better knows the problems at a worksite than the people on the job every day? Input from workers will ensure that policies and control measures are relevant to actual work conditions. Furthermore, workers may identify problems in the workplace that managers and others may overlook. Credibility and acceptance of TB programs is enhanced when rank and file workers have a voice in decision-making. Moreover, when workers are represented by a collective bargaining agent, union representation should be included in developing TB control programs. Engaging workers in a TB task force will provide a process that incorporates workers' concerns and ideas into the planning of prevention programs, including educational programs, as they are developed.

Conducting a needs assessment is critical to developing a training program. One method is to run focus groups composed of affected workers. Focus groups can help identify the knowledge that workers already have, problems they perceive, and information they need. For a focus group to be productive, the facilitator should not dominate the discussion but keep the participants relaxed and engaged in discussing their concerns. This method encourages broad participation and can be useful in developing an appropriate agenda for future training sessions.

Well-designed training programs will delineate steps that must be accomplished by individuals, institutions, and government to combat TB.

As individuals, workers may need to comply with respiratory protection programs, participate in a medical surveillance program, report suspected cases of TB, and ensure that TB controls are in place (i.e., keeping isolation room doors closed). On a personal level, they need to learn about risk factors that can increase their susceptibility to developing active TB if they are already infected.

On an institutional or agency level, a proper TB control plan contains numerous facets, including early identification and isolation, improving environmental controls, providing personal protective equipment where appropriate, implementing workplace screening programs, and developing suitable and effective education programs. Site-specific control measures implemented at an institution or agency should be explained in training programs. A proactive approach to TB control on an institutional level is obviously preferable to reacting to a nosocomial outbreak or orders from an enforcement agency.

Implementation of workplace policies and regulations requires a knowledgeable workforce. Although OSHA issued a national enforcement policy and procedure for occupational exposure to TB[20] in October 1993, enforcement may be modest. In many social service settings, the regulations may not even apply. These circumstances increase the need for greater reliance on worker knowledge to ensure workplace safety.

WHO NEEDS TB EDUCATION?

Workers in many different occupational settings need to learn about tuberculosis, but government agencies have narrowly defined the worksites where TB training programs are required. The CDC has published reports and recommendations for the control of TB in health care settings (hospitals, emergency medical services, autopsy rooms, home health services, and outpatient clinics),[5,12] correctional institutions, including police lockups,[4] homeless shelters,[3] long-term care facilities,[6] and drug treatment centers.[8] Consequently, only workers in these facilities are considered to be at "high risk" by the CDC, OSHA,[20,21] CalOSHA,[16] and the New York State Department of Labor (covering New York public employees),[15] therefore requiring education about the disease.

In addition to the work settings listed above, occupational exposure to TB may also affect criminal justice workers, school teachers, and employees in many social service agencies located in geographic areas where there are high rates of TB. Agencies providing services to people with AIDS and to homeless people should be particularly concerned about TB. TB education, specifically the occupational health aspects, should also be included in the training of all health professionals (e.g., nurses, x-ray technicians, and laboratory technologists). In addition to protecting the health of these workers, training will also increase their capacity to contribute to TB prevention among the clients they serve.

ELEMENTS OF TB TRAINING PROGRAMS

Although worksite education programs may emphasize different aspects, the basic elements of a worker-oriented TB training program include the following:

1. **History and reemergence of TB.** In a discussion of these issues, workers learn about the socioeconomic conditions that promote the spread of TB. An examination of conditions at the beginning of this century, including tenement living, 14-hour work days, lack of health care, poor nutrition, and widespread poverty, provides a perspective on the socioeconomic roots of TB. When discussing the current reemergence of TB, it is important to examine socioeconomic factors, including homelessness, poverty, drug use, and the decreased availability of health care and nutrition programs.

2. **Epidemiology: Who has TB?** An analytical look at the populations that are developing TB will illuminate the important role that social conditions and HIV play in the spread of the disease.

3. **Transmission of disease.** The emphasis in this section should be on the airborne nature of transmission and the difference between TB infection and disease. Worksite training programs should present current scientific knowledge on TB transmission and progression to active disease.

4. **Diagnosis of tuberculosis.** A TB training program should include a discussion of the tools used to diagnose TB, including the role of skin testing,

symptomatology, chest x-rays, examination of sputum smears, and culturing the sputum. Factors that complicate the diagnosis also should be specified. An adequate understanding of these issues is important to allow workers to protect themselves and to play a role in the administrative controls of early diagnosis and treatment.[12]

5. Medical surveillance and prophylaxis (PPD testing). Policies on PPD testing of workers and patients should be reviewed in a training session. Skin testing helps to identify infected patients for follow-up treatment and care. In some cases, a program of preventive drug therapy is recommended to reduce the likelihood of progression to active disease. A review of PPD test conversion rates and follow-up action should also be covered. Workers need to understand the usefulness of PPD testing in detecting infection and implementing a prevention program, the limitations of PPD testing for people with compromised immune systems, and the role of bacille Calmette-Guérin (BCG) vaccine.

The BCG vaccine, although used in different forms all over the world, is limited in its effectiveness. While some forms of the vaccine protect against TB, immunity tends to decrease with time. In addition, not all BCG vaccines are equally effective in stopping the progression of disease. Because of the variability and unreliability of BCG vaccines, the CDC recommends that workers who have received these vaccines should not be excluded from a skin-testing program.

6. Treatment of TB. Including this topic in a training program enables workers to play a vital role in patients' treatment as well as in their own therapy if they become infected or develop active tuberculosis. The increased incidence of multidrug-resistant TB is directly related to patients' noncompliance with drug therapies. This topic can be addressed by engaging workers in discussions of the factors involved in patients' compliance with medications so that they can help ensure that patients complete their drug therapy. Additionally, institutions that provide directly observed therapy should stress the importance of these programs in training sessions.

7. Multidrug-resistant TB. A discussion of MDR-TB should include (1) what it is—TB bacilli that continue to grow in the presence of antiTB medication; (2) how it evolves—primary drug resistance occurs when a person is infected by drug-resistant TB, and secondary resistance can occur when a person with TB disease stops taking prescribed medications or when a physician fails to monitor and treat patients with appropriate drugs; and (3) the importance of TB patients taking drugs as prescribed.

8. TB and HIV: How TB affects people living with HIV and AIDS and other immunocompromising conditions. It is necessary to include this topic in a workplace education program for a number of reasons: Workers who are infected with HIV need to know about their own risks; institutions need to develop policies for immunocompromised workers; and health workers who treat patients with immunocompromising conditions such as HIV and AIDS need to be alert to the patient's increased risk of developing active disease if the patient also is infected with TB. Training should also address negative attitudes toward people with HIV, since these attitudes are also often held toward patients with TB.

9. TB prevention. TB education is most meaningful when it is presented in the context of a workplace prevention and control program. Training workers on site-specific components of a TB control plan is essential to protecting workers and patients alike. For example, in a hospital, training should cover the facility's procedures for reporting suspect cases, the location of isolation rooms and how negative pressure is maintained, the proper selection and use of personal protective equipment and where it can be procured, and TB screening protocol and its effectiveness. Discussing preventive measures in a training session may also serve to identify deficiencies in current controls and obtain input from participants on possible solutions. A site-specific hands-on approach to training should help improve employee participation in screening programs, reporting suspect cases of TB, maintaining engineering controls such as keeping isolation room doors closed, and using personal protective equipment such as respirators.

The topics listed above outline the basic elements of a TB education program. In addition to covering specific topics, training should be presented to employees upon hire and annually thereafter to provide updated information. Training should always be done on work time. Table 1 contains the CDC's recommendations for health care worker training and education on TB.

TRAINING METHODOLOGY

Training programs that actively engage workers will be most effective in achieving improvements in the workplace. These programs should emphasize knowledge and skills development. For example, using case studies to teach how to identify suspect cases, demonstrating proper use of personal protective equipment, and demonstrating how to check negative air pressure are effective training methods.

According to Wallerstein and Rubenstein, "An education session will work best if participants have the opportunity to engage in multiple-learning modalities: to listen, look at visuals, ask questions, simulate situations, read, write, practice with equipment, and discuss critical issues. If the goal of an educational session is

TABLE 1. CDC Recommended Guidelines on Training and Education of Health Care Workers on Tuberculosis

Training should be appropriate to a health care worker's job category and should be conducted before initial assignment and annually. The following elements should be included in the training of all health care workers.

- The basic concepts of TB transmission, pathogenesis, and diagnosis
- The risk of occupational exposure to people with infectious TB in the health care facility, including the prevalence of TB in the community and facility and the ability of the facility to use correct isolation procedures
- Principles and practices of infection control that reduce the risk of transmission of TB, including the written policy of the facility and any site-specific control measures
- The purpose of PPD testing and significance of positive results
- Effectiveness and side effects of preventive therapy for TB infection
- Workers' responsibility for medical evaluation if symptoms develop or PPD conversion occurs
- Principles of drug therapy for active TB
- Notification of facility when active TB occurs so contact investigation can begin
- Facility's maintenance of confidentiality of workers with active TB while providing treatment
- Higher risk to immunocompromised individuals, including discussion of drug-resistant TB
- Potential development of cutaneous anergy as immune function declines
- Facility's policy on voluntary work reassignment options

From Centers for Disease Control and Prevention: Draft guidelines for preventing the transmission of tuberculosis in health care facilities, 2nd ed. Notice of comment period. Federal Register 58:52810–52854, October 12, 1993.

for workers to take actions to improve their health and safety, then sessions must involve workers in critical thinking, identification of problems, planning social actions and trying out strategies in participatory ways."[22]

Lectures, videos, and self-tests can be a useful part of a TB training but should only be used along with participatory activities. There is a commonly expressed belief among health educators that people learn 20% of what they hear, 40% of what they read, 60% of what they read and hear, and 80% of what they read, hear, and do.

Because issues in a TB training are very complex, participants are likely to learn more when classes are limited to fewer than 20 participants. Small class size maximizes the opportunity for participation in activities that reinforce information and allow workers to interact informally and learn from each other.

In the experience of NYCOSH and PEF, workers learn more when engaged in small group activities than when in traditional classes. Using the small group activity method, trainees form groups of 4–6 and are asked to solve problems related to TB using their own experience and knowledge along with written materials or case studies.

Hands-on exercises are the most effective training method. For example, a demonstration of how to use a smoke tube to check an isolation room for negative air pressure is far more effective than an explanation of how it is done.

In worksites that have not begun to address TB, health educators, unions, and advocacy groups can provide training to educate and motivate workers and employers to develop full TB prevention programs. The small group activity described in the box on this page may be used in such instances.

The most effective training programs of this kind will inspire the development of concrete action plans.

Developing a Worksite TB Prevention and Control Program

Each agency needs to determine what is appropriate and possible for inclusion in its workplace TB program. In this activity, divide the participants into groups of four or five. You can provide copies of TB guidelines from the CDC, OSHA, and your state. *Briefly* go over the key components of a workplace program. Describe each one with a few sentences without going into great detail—that's the job of the participants in each small group. As you introduce each element of a workplace program, list them on the flip chart. Give each group 30–40 minutes to perform the following tasks:

Task 1
- Choose the three most important elements of a workplace program for your agency. (The group will discuss all of the elements and try to reach a consensus on which are the three most important.) Tell participants to be prepared to explain their choices.

Task 2
- For each of the three elements in your program, do the following:
  a. List issues that may affect employees, volunteers, or clients by implementing this measure.
  b. List the resources that are needed to implement items, i.e., for TB screening you will need to identify a screening site and a centralized, confidential system to keep all records.
  c. Determine what agencies can help you put this component of the program in place.
  d. List the obstacles to implementation.
  e. List ideas on how you can overcome these barriers.

Have each group report back to the large group, eliciting comments from the others.

In sites that employ large numbers of workers, consideration should be given to developing a train-the-trainer program, thus reducing the reliance on outside educators. Carefully crafted and monitored train-the-trainer programs can promote further worker involvement. Unions, employers, and occupational and public health advocates can collaborate on the development of joint programs using a train-the-trainer approach.

DESIGNING TRAINING FOR SPECIFIC WORKPLACES

In all settings, workers should be involved in the development of a worksite TB program, including the training. In unionized worksites, workers usually have a greater opportunity for input into the content of health and safety programs. Unions provide an existing mechanism for employee involvement, e.g., through labor-management meetings (see box on page 689).

As with all worker training, the content of a TB education program should be tailored to reflect the actual issues at the worksite. For instance, in the PEF/New York State Division of Parole program, information on isolation rooms and personal protective equipment is deemphasized since the division does not provide medical care. Instead, emphasis is placed on reviewing the division's policy guidelines on staff monitoring of releasees with TB. These guidelines specify actions parole officers should take when parolees are exhibiting TB symptoms, are on TB medications, or have active TB disease. The mode of training will also need to be specific to the organizational culture, resources, and special needs of each workplace.

Small community-based organizations, such as drug treatment centers and small shelters that serve client populations with high rates of TB, often lack the funds and expertise to institute comprehensive TB control programs. Even large hospitals and government agencies are under significant fiscal pressure. When developing TB education programs it is important to consider these obstacles and incorporate innovative strategies for overcoming them.

HIV/AIDS service agencies should emphasize the risk of TB to both clients and workers who are HIV-infected. Workers with HIV or AIDS or other immunocompromising conditions who are exposed to TB should be informed of the dangers presented by the disease and should be given the option of reassignment. In fact, all workers who are exposed to TB are at risk of developing infection, and this risk must be conveyed in a training program. But because people who are immunocompromised have an increased risk of developing active disease if infected, they need additional protection.

OBSTACLES TO EFFECTIVE WORKPLACE TB EDUCATION

While each worksite may face its own unique set of obstacles, some general points are applicable to most places.

1. For engineering controls to be even potentially effective, they must be properly installed, operated, and maintained. Many controls require extensive education for proper use. Ultraviolet lights, for example, can harm workers maintaining them and others in the area unless they are properly installed and maintained. Ventilation systems can be rendered ineffective if not maintained. Proper training should include basic information on how each control measure operates and how it must be maintained.

2. Regulations and guidelines that govern workplace exposures to TB are confusing, and conflicting, or nonexistent. Guidelines from the CDC, state and city departments of health, federal OSHA, state OSHA plans, and NIOSH provide

A Model TB Education Program: The Partnership between The New York State Public Employees Federation and The New York State Division of Parole

In 1991, after a number of prisoners and a corrections officer in the New York state prison system died from an outbreak of multidrug-resistant tuberculosis, the Public Employees Federation (PEF) and the Division of Parole began an ambitious program to educate and screen all 2,000 employees within the division.

New York state parole officers supervise state prison releasees. The Department of Correctional Services screening program indicates that 25% of the inmates have latent TB infection. There were 116 active TB cases among 65,000 inmates in 1992.

Union representatives had been raising concerns about tuberculosis to management for 6 months prior to the reported outbreak, but a consensus on control measures was not achieved. Subsequently, the state health department, in an effort to address the concerns of employees and management, issued *An Action Plan for Controlling TB* in the Division of Parole. As a first step, the chairman of the parole board asked the union leadership to participate in a joint tuberculosis task force. Participants from management included representatives from human resources, staff development, and client services. Union representatives were from the joint health and safety committee and included PEF's health and safety specialist. Together, a two-pronged plan was developed to screen every parole employee and implement an education program.

A massive screening program was conducted at multiple sites around the state. At the union's suggestion, health educators were present at each of the skin-testing sites, allowing workers to obtain information and get questions answered on the spot. Employees testing positive received private counseling on workers' compensation, a reiteration of the basic information on TB infection and disease, and information on the importance of obtaining follow-up medical evaluation. TB factsheets and *Parole TB Guidelines* were provided for all employees.

Working together, PEF and the Division of Parole developed a curriculum for training trainers within the division to conduct TB education programs statewide. The curriculum was reviewed by experts from CDC, the state health department, the American Lung Association, and others. The program features multiple training modalities, including small group activities and the use of overhead transparencies and handouts. Trainers were jointly selected by the union and management and included volunteers with a strong interest in TB training as well as workers whose jobs include training responsibilities. A full-day train-the-trainer session attended by 10 parole officers included practice sessions in which participants used the curriculum to practice delivery of the module.

Experts from state agencies, other unions, COSH groups, and community organizations were invited to these sessions and have subsequently been called upon to assist in training sessions around the state.

Since this initial training, the trainers—PEF members and parole management—have conducted 2–3 hour educational sessions throughout the division. More than 1,500 parole employees were trained over a 7-month period. The union has benefited from this strategy because members receive quality training, often from peers. The employer benefits because in-house resources are used at low cost. Both parties take pride in ownership of a program developed jointly, and the program is relevant to the needs of the workers since it was developed by people who are part of the agency and know its work and organizational culture.

A policy on staff/releasee contact was also developed that provides guidance to parole officers in monitoring releasees' TB status and ensuring that proper steps are taken to protect the health of releasees and parole staff.

The outcome of this program is a high level of awareness of TB within the division. Furthermore, compliance with the parole skin-testing program is extremely high. By training trainers, a pool of people are now in place to act as worksite resources.

In conclusion, the efforts to monitor releasees' TB status ultimately will allow parole employees to make an important contribution to fighting TB as well as protecting their own health.

conflicting recommendations. Confusion also exists over what is an enforceable regulation versus recommended guideline, and which entities have legal jurisdiction. With the issuance of CDC's guidelines and OSHA's national enforcement policies and procedures, the confusion may be lessened.

When federal guidelines contradict regional regulations, institutions will often comply with the least expensive or restrictive. Conflicting guidelines, such as those for respiratory protection, have led to institutional gridlock. Workers can become confused by this overlapping web of guidelines.

Many social service settings do not fall under the jurisdiction of any of the regulations regarding workplace TB exposure, leading to inaction on the part of some agencies.

3. Prejudice, fear, mistrust, and misinformation present obstacles to understanding TB, just as they did with HIV and AIDS. Tendencies to blame the resurgence of TB on groups with the highest rates of the disease, including blacks and Hispanics, homeless people, and people with HIV should be addressed. One of the goals of training should be to replace victim-blaming stereotypes with facts about the disease.

4. Racist attitudes can hinder the ability to learn about TB and, consequently, to take appropriate actions. Because people living in communities with the fewest social services and the highest rates of poverty, unemployment, and homelessness are often black or Hispanic, racism can become a serious obstacle to understanding the real causes of the spread of TB. Trainers should recognize and address the attitudes and biases that interfere with understanding TB. Effective training can reduce workers' fears related to tuberculosis.

5. Meeting the demands for workplace safety and health while simultaneously protecting clients' and workers' rights to confidentiality can be difficult. The identity of a worker with active TB may be revealed to those who have had direct contact with him or her. While contact tracing is important for workers' health, it may violate confidentiality. This becomes even further complicated when a patient or worker who has developed TB disease has HIV infection. As we learned with HIV, workers' "right to know" is often at odds with patients' and other workers' rights to confidentiality.

6. An agency's ability to effect specific changes is largely dependent on its finances. The action plan and educational component should reflect the realistic funds that a workplace can commit. An agency's financial situation may present a real obstacle to putting changes in place, and the training should reflect this reality. In so doing, false expectations will not be raised.

7. The importance of TB education is underrecognized. Institutions developing TB prevention programs, such as hospitals and correctional facilities, have focused most of their attention on skin testing, upgrading isolation rooms, and instituting a respiratory protection program. In general, there is a lack of recognition of the role education plays in TB prevention, resulting in few or limited training programs. The 1993 CDC draft guidelines include references to the need for education: "Implementation of a minimum TB control program requires risk assessment; early identification and isolation of infectious TB patients; effective engineering controls; an appropriate respiratory protection program; *and health care worker TB education,* counseling, screening and evaluation."[12] (Emphasis added.)

8. Organizations suffer from a lack of employee involvement. Institutions that do not involve workers in the design of TB control programs may achieve limited results and experience reduced effectiveness and credibility.

In conclusion, it is clear that the rising TB epidemic requires a long-term commitment of public and private health resources. Training and education on an annual basis must become a key component of the commitment of employers, labor, and government. Clearly, an educated workforce can play a central role in TB control efforts for patients and staff.

RESOURCES FOR EDUCATION

Educational programs and training curricula that have been developed from an occupational health perspective can be obtained from the following groups:

New York Committee for Occupational Safety and Health (NYCOSH)

NYCOSH, one of 25 COSH (Committees for Occupational Safety and Health) groups nationwide, is a coalition of labor unions and occupational safety and health professionals and activists providing worker training programs. NYCOSH has been training workers for more than 13 years and in the past 3 years has developed an extensive TB program for various unions. In addition, NYCOSH's technical staff has consulted with unions and employers on ventilation systems in hospitals and offices where there is a risk of TB transmission.

New York State Public Employees Federation (see box on page 689.)

One of NYCOSH's member unions is the New York State Public Employees Federation (PEF), representing 55,000 professional, scientific, and technical state employees. PEF designed, developed, and implemented a model statewide TB education program with the New York State Division of Parole for its 2,000 employees. Revised versions of the curriculum are being used by the NYS Department of Correctional Services to train its 30,000 employees, and the NYS Office of Mental Health's 28,000 workers.

Hunter College Center on AIDS, Drugs, and Community Health

This center in New York City has provided AIDS education to agencies serving HIV-infected clients for the past 6 years. Hunter's TB training program and curriculum arose from a need expressed by AIDS agencies to protect their clients and staff from this new epidemic. In addition to conducting educational programs in shelters, prisons, AIDS housing projects, and drug treatment centers, the Hunter program has held seminars for administrators of AIDS agencies to discuss the development of a comprehensive TB program. Working with the Hunter College Center on Occupational and Environmental Health, the AIDS center produced a worksite assessment manual for use by small service agencies.

RESOURCE GUIDE

Below is a listing of various agencies and organizations that can be contacted for information on tuberculosis.

Government Agencies

National

U.S. Department of Labor
Occupational Safety and Health Administration
Washington, DC 20210
(202) 219-8021—Call for regional and area offices

Centers for Disease Control
Information Services
1600 Clifton Road, NE, Mailstop E-06
Atlanta, GA 30333
(404) 332-4555 (recording)
(404) 639-3311 (switchboard)

National Institute for Occupational Safety and Health (NIOSH)
4676 Columbia Parkway
Cincinnati, OH 45226
(800) 356-4674

Health Departments

Contact your state, county, or municipal health departments for information and training on tuberculosis.

Tuberculosis Training Organizations

Hunter College Center on AIDS, Drugs, and Community Health
425 East 25th Street
New York, NY 10010
(212) 481-7672

Hunter College Center on Occupational and Environmental Health
425 East 25th Street
New York, NY 10010
(212) 481-4361

New York Committee for Occupational Safety and Health
275 Seventh Avenue
New York, NY 10001
(212) 627-3900

Labor Occupational Health Program
2515 Channing Way
Berkeley, CA 94720
(510) 642-5507

Western Massachusetts Committee on Occupational Safety and Health
458 Bridge Street
Springfield, MA 01103
(413) 731-0760

The Labor Institute
853 Broadway
New York, NY 10003
(212) 674-3322

Unions Providing TB Educational Materials and Training

American Federation of State, County, and Municipal Employees (AFSCME)
Safety and Health Department
1625 L Street, NW
Washington, DC 20036
(202) 429-1000

American Federation of Teachers
Safety and Health Department
555 New Jersey Avenue, NW
Washington, DC 20001
(202) 393-5674

District Council 37, AFSCME
125 Barclay Street
New York, NY 10007
(212) 815-1685

Local 1199, Health Care and Human Service Employees Union
310 West 43rd Street
New York, NY 10036
(212) 582-1890

New York State Public Employees Federation
Safety and Health Program
1168-70 Troy-Schenectady Road
P.O. Box 2414
Albany, NY 12212-2414
(518) 785-1900, ext. 254

Service Employees International Union
Safety and Health Department
1313 L Street NW
Washington, DC 20005
(202) 898-3200

Voluntary Agencies
American Lung Association
1740 Broadway
New York, NY 10019
(212) 315-8700

The American Lung Association has affiliates all over the country. Check your local phone book for listings in your area. Most affiliates provide written material and training services on tuberculosis.

REFERENCES

1. At least 17 health care workers developed active multidrug-resistant TB, CDC official says. Occupational Safety and Health Reporter, Bureau of National Affairs, February 3, 1993.
2. Blood-lead levels dropped, knowledge improved after implementation of health education plan. Occupational Safety and Health Reporter, Bureau of National Affairs, March 10, 1993.
3. Centers for Disease Control: Tuberculosis control among homeless populations. MMWR 36, May 8, 1987.
4. Centers for Disease Control: Prevention and control of tuberculosis in correctional institutions: Recommendations of the Advisory Committee for the Elimination of Tuberculosis. MMWR 38:313–320, 325, 1989.
5. Centers for Disease Control: Guidelines for preventing the transmission of tuberculosis in health-care settings, with special focus on HIV-related issues. MMWR 39(RR-17):1–28, 1990.
6. Centers for Disease Control: Prevention and control of tuberculosis in facilities providing long-term care to the elderly: Recommendations of the Advisory Committee for the Elimination of Tuberculosis. MMWR 39(RR-10):7–13, 1990.
7. Centers for Disease Control: Core Curriculum on Tuberculosis. Atlanta, Centers for Disease Control, April 1991.
8. Centers for Disease Control: Transmission of multidrug-resistant tuberculosis from an HIV-positive client in a residential substance-abuse treatment facility—Michigan. MMWR 40(RR-8):129–131, 1991.
9. Centers for Disease Control: Transmission of multidrug-resistant tuberculosis among immuno-compromised persons in a correctional system—New York, 1991. MMWR 41, July 17, 1992.
10. Centers for Disease Control: Initial therapy for tuberculosis in the era of multidrug resistance: Recommendations of the Advisory Committee for the Elimination of Tuberculosis. MMWR 42(RR-7):1–8, 1993.
11. Centers for Disease Control: Probable transmission of multidrug-resistant tuberculosis in a correctional facility—California. MMWR 42, January 29, 1993.
12. Centers for Disease Control and Prevention: Draft guidelines for preventing the transmission of tuberculosis in health care facilities, 2nd ed; Notice of comment period. Federal Register 58:52810–52854, October 12, 1993.
13. Coughlin TA III: Press release. State of New York Department of Correctional Services, Novermber 15, 1991.
14. Guanay W: An outbreak of multiple-drug resistant tuberculosis among New York State correctional facility inmates. New York State Commission of Correction, Medical Review Board, Special Report, July 1992.
15. New York State Department of Labor: Enforcement guidelines for occupational exposure to tuberculosis. Albany, April 7, 1992.

16. Occupational tuberculosis control: Section 5197, Title 8, California Code of Regulations, Division 1, Chapter 4, Subchapter 7, Group 16, Control of Hazardous Substances and Processes (draft 1). December 21, 1992.
17. Pearson ML, Jereb JA, Frieden TR, et al: Nosocomial transmission of multiple drug resistant Mycobacterium tuberculosis: A risk to patients and health care workers. Ann Intern Med 117:191–196, 1992.
18. TB conversion rate as high as 50 percent in workers caring for infected patients: Study. Occupational Safety and Health Reporter, Bureau of National Affairs, August 5, 1992.
19. TB conversions continue despite controls, according to early results from NIOSH report. Occupational Safety and Health Reporter, Bureau of National Affairs, October 28, 1992.
20. U.S. Department of Labor, Occupational Safety and Health Administration: Enforcement policy and procedures for occupational exposure to tuberculosis; memorandum to regional administrators. October 8, 1993.
21. U.S. Department of Labor, Occupational Safety and Health Administration, Region II: Enforcement guidelines for occupational exposure to tuberculosis. May 7, 1992.
22. Wallerstein N, Rubenstein H: Teaching About Job Hazards: A Guide for Workers and Their Providers. Washington, DC, American Public Health Association, 1993.

JACQUELINE M. MOLINE, MD, MSc
STEVEN B. MARKOWITZ, MD

MEDICAL SURVEILLANCE FOR WORKERS EXPOSED TO TUBERCULOSIS

From the Division of Environmental and Occupational Medicine
Mount Sinai School of Medicine
New York, New York

Reprint requests to:
Jacqueline M. Moline, MD, MSc
Division of Environmental and Occupational Medicine
Mount Sinai School of Medicine
1 Gustave L. Levy Place
New York, NY 10029

"The most critical element in tuberculosis elimination is the detection and treatment of infected persons before disease emerges," according to the Centers of Disease Control and Prevention.[9] The challenge implicit in the statement is daunting yet vital. Currently, an estimated 10 million people in the United States[15] and more than 2 billion people worldwide are infected with *Mycobacterium tuberculosis*.[50] Ninety percent of all new cases of tuberculosis in the United States arise from this group of already infected individuals. Surveillance programs, including those in the workplace, can identify many of these individuals and, with proper treatment, can lessen the spread of infection both in and out of the work environment.

The decreased incidence of tuberculosis in the United States as a whole compared to three or four decades ago has made routine screening of the general population inefficient. It is important to recognize that certain groups of individuals may have higher incidence rates of infection because "the group may have a higher prevalence of infection or the group may have a higher risk of disease for any given prevalence of infection."[11]

The CDC's Advisory Committee for the Elimination of Tuberculosis (ACET) recommends that the following groups be included in screening programs for active tuberculosis disease and latent tuberculosis infection:[11]

- People infected with the human immunodeficiency virus (HIV)

- Close contacts of people known or suspected to have tuberculosis, sharing the same household or other enclosed environments
- People with medical risk factors known to increase the risk of disease if infection has occurred
- Foreign-born people from countries with a high prevalence of TB
- Medically underserved low-income populations, including high-risk racial or ethnic minority populations such as blacks, Hispanics, and Native Americans
- Alcoholics and intravenous drug users
- Residents of long-term care facilities, correctional institutions, mental institutions, nursing homes, and other long-term residential facilities

Among the groups of people for whom screening is recommended are those that work in occupations that entail significant exposure to persons with active tuberculosis. The CDC specifically recommends TB screening programs for workers who are employed in health care settings, correctional institutions, homeless shelters, long-term care facilities for the elderly, and drug treatment centers.[10,12,19,25] It is also reasonable to institute TB surveillance programs for workers in related settings that serve or assist the same people who use the institutions specified above. These settings include social service, housing, and other organizations that help people who have an increased risk of active TB.

Knowledge of nonoccupational risk factors for TB is also important in the design and implementation of proper workplace TB surveillance programs. The prevalence of tuberculosis is highest among elderly people, prison inmates, homeless people, alcoholics, people who inject drugs, immigrants from countries with high rates of TB, and selected segments of minority populations, including black Americans, Hispanics, Asians, and Native Americans.[25]

Like all medical screening programs, the usefulness of a TB screening program depends on its ability to satisfy certain criteria, including the use of sensitive and specific tests, low cost, availability of technology and skill, and the existence of effective intervention.[77]

The hallmark of an effective surveillance program is the ability to identify individuals infected with tuberculosis before they develop active disease. As with any screening or surveillance program, it is essential to ensure that proper follow-up occurs after any screening activities and that the appropriate administration of preventive therapy receives as high a priority as screening.

THE TUBERCULIN SKIN TEST

The tuberculin skin test in use today is considered to be the simplest and most accurate method of detecting tuberculosis infection. Indeed, it is the only method currently available for demonstrating latent infection with *M. tuberculosis.* This skin test is based on a method developed in the late 19th century by Robert Koch. Unfortunately, a better method for detecting latent tuberculosis in the general population has not yet arisen. The skin test is based on the fact that infection with *M. tuberculosis* produces sensitivity to certain components of this organism, or antigens, which are contained in culture extracts known as tuberculins. The reaction to injected tuberculin is a classic manifestation of a delayed hypersensitivity reaction. An intact immune system is essential for the development of a positive skin reaction. Any impairment of the cell-mediated immune response may result in a false negative skin test. The proper technique must also be used in the administration and reading of the tuberculin skin test in order for it to have any degree of validity. An additional factor essential for the proper interpretation of a positive skin test is recent local epidemiologic and clinical experiences with the test. Proper use and interpretation of the skin test depends on the integration of all these factors.

The Components of the Skin Test

Two licensed tuberculin preparations are available for use in the United States: old tuberculin (OT) and purified protein derivative (PPD). OT is a filtrate prepared from heat-sterilized, concentrated broth cultures of tubercle bacilli. Produced in the 19th century by Koch, this substance was initially used as a treatment for tuberculosis infection but proved to be ineffective. OT is only available for use in multiple puncture devices. PPD, originally made in 1934 by Florence Siebert, is a protein precipitate obtained from filtrates of OT after heat-concentration and separation with trichloroacetic acid. A large batch of PPD was produced by Siebert in 1939 and designated PPD-S. This batch was prepared for use as the standard tuberculin preparation in the United States and remains the standard to the present.[33]

The standard skin test of 5 tuberculin units (TU) of PPD-S is defined as the delayed skin test activity contained in a 0.1 μg/0.1 mL dose of PPD-S. The standard test dose of a commercial PPD preparation is defined as the dose that yields biological activity equivalent to 5 TU of PPD-S (i.e., it elicits reactions of equivalent size within a 20% range). All PPD products currently licensed must meet these criteria. Preparations of 1 TU and 250 TU are also on the market. These contain one fifth and 50 times, respectively, the concentration of antigen determined to be bioequivalent to 5 TU PPD-S, but are not considered to be useful in diagnosing tuberculosis infection. The 250 TU product is sometimes used to assess a patient's immunologic status.[3]

Certain precautions must be taken in the handling of PPD in order to ensure consistent test conditions. A detergent, Tween 80, is added by tuberculin manufacturers to all preparations to reduce adsorption of the protein to containers or tubing. To minimize the reduction in potency due to adsorption, tuberculin should never be transferred from one container to another. Skin tests should be given as soon as possible after the syringe has been filled. The test dose should be kept refrigerated until use, and it should be removed from the vial under aseptic conditions. Tuberculin should be kept away from direct light and kept in the dark as much as possible.[33] In the past, false positive reactions occured after several employees in a screening program had a "positive" reaction with an atypical appearance after using Aplisol (Parke-Davis). The results were not confirmed when another brand, Tubersol (Connaught), was used. The lot of Aplisol associated with the atypical reaction was removed from the market, and there have been no similar problems since a new batch was made.[4,49]

Administration of the Skin Test

The Mantoux skin test involves the administration of an intracutaneous injection of 0.1 mL of 5 TU of PPD into either the volar or dorsal surface of the forearm. This should be placed in a skin area free of lesions or veins. The injection is made with a short (¼- to ½-inch) bluntly beveled platinum or steel needle, with a gauge of 26 or 27, and a glass or plastic tuberculin syringe. The injection should be made just beneath the surface of the skin and placed with the bevel of the needle upward. A discrete pale elevation of the skin (a wheal) should be produced after the tuberculin has been injected intracutaneously. If a wheal is not evident or there is concern whether the skin test has been placed properly, another test dose can be given immediately several centimeters away from the original injection site.[33]

The PPD skin tests should be read 48–72 hours after injection. The skin test must be read by a trained individual, and under no circumstance (including the testing of health care workers) should patients be allowed to read the test themselves. A study of healthy volunteers found that only 37% of those with a positive PPD were able to correctly identify that induration was present. Conversely, five volunteers stated that induration was present when none was palpated by an examiner.[43]

The skin test should be read by a trained professional in a good light, with the forearm slightly flexed at the elbow. The basis of the reading is the presence or absence of induration, not erythema, and is determined by both inspection and palpation. The transverse diameter of induration should be recorded in millimeters. Another method of reading skin tests has been described in the literature: the pen method. Using the pen method, the interpreter draws a line with a medium ball-point pen toward the center from a point 1–2 cm away from the margin of the skin test reaction. The pen is moved slowly, and when it reaches the margin of the indurated area, definite resistance to further movement is noted and the pen is lifted. The procedure is repeated from the opposite side of the reaction. The lines drawn by the pen provide a visible record of the margins of induration, which can then be quantified.[69] While some authors state that the pen method can lead to a substantial reduction in observer variation of skin test reactions,[69] others feel that pen measurements must be interpreted with caution.[43]

The variability in the performance and interpretation of the skin test has been recognized as an important problem in tuberculosis testing. In a study of healthy volunteers who had two simultaneously placed skin tests read by trained personnel, the examiners agreed about 68% of the time. In volunteers with bacteriologically confirmed tuberculosis, the agreement rose to 87%.[26] Another study found that observers agreed in 98% of cases in a comparison of the Mantoux and tine tests. The false negative rate for the Mantoux test in this study was identified as 5%, which the authors attributed to the difficulty of accurate intradermal injection, even for experienced practitioners.[61]

Multiple puncture devices containing OT or PPD introduce tuberculin into the skin either by puncture with an applicator with points coated with dried tuberculin into the skin or by puncture through a film of liquid tuberculin. With this delivery system, the quantity of tuberculin actually introduced into the skin cannot be controlled. For these reasons, multiple puncture devices are not recommended by the American Thoracic Society or the CDC for use in tuberculosis screening programs.[15,33] Any positive test result obtained with a multiple puncture device should be verified with a Mantoux skin test.

Adverse reactions after the administration of the purified protein derivative are unusual and do not increase the size of induration. The most common adverse reaction is an immediate hypersensitivity reaction to tuberculin or constituents of the diluents. It usually begins shortly after the skin injection and disappears by 24 hours.[33,41] The reaction consists mainly of vesicle formation and/or local induration at the injection site and, more rarely, fever and lymphadenopathy. No specific therapy except for a topical agent such as petroleum jelly is indicated.[41] The use of a lower-strength dosage (1 TU) of PPD does not affect the intensity of these immediate reactions and are not recommended in such rare individuals.

Reaction to the Skin Test

The reaction to injected tuberculin is a classic example of a delayed hypersensitivity reaction. The reaction has a delayed course, reaching a peak more than 24 hours after injection and has an indurated character due to local cell infiltration. The reaction measures the immune response of the host to the actual bacilli, rather than a reaction from a toxin or other product of the bacteria. The hypersensitivity to components of the tubercle bacillus, as is demonstrated by the development of a skin reaction, is detectable 2–10 weeks after infection with *M. tuberculosis,* which corresponds to the time needed to develop a cell-mediated immune response.[3]

Many factors can cause a decreased ability to respond to tuberculin, since the generation and maintenance of a tuberculosis reaction in people infected with tubercle bacillus requires a complex interaction of immunologic responses[33] (Table 1). Up to 30% of patients with human immunodeficiency virus (HIV) and 60% of patients with acquired immunodeficiency syndrome (AIDS) may have skin reactions of less than 5 mm induration even though they are infected with tubercle bacilli.[15] In addition, up to 25% of people with fulminant tuberculosis will not have a significant skin test reaction.[6] However, the existence of a condition or factor that is associated with a failure to respond to the skin test should not deter the individual from having a tuberculin skin test, nor should it be considered a

TABLE 1. Factors Causing Decreased Ability to Respond to Tuberculin

Factors Related to the Person Tested
- Infections
  - viral (measles, mumps, chickenpox, HIV)
  - bacterial (typhoid fever, brucellosis, typhus, leprosy, pertussis, overwhelming tuberculosis, tuberculous pleurisy)
  - fungal (South American blastomycosis)
- Live virus vaccinations (measles, mumps, polio)
- Metabolic derangements (chronic renal failure)
- Nutritional factors (severe protein deficiency)
- Diseases affecting lymphoid organs (Hodgkin's disease, lymphoma, chronic lymphocytic leukemia, sarcoidosis)
- Drugs (corticosteroids and many other immunosuppressive agents)
- Age (newborns, elderly patients with "waned" sensitivity)
- Recent or overwhelming infection with *M. tuberculosis*
- Stress (surgery, burns, mental illness, graft versus host reaction)

Factors Related to the Test Itself
- Improper storage of the tuberculin (exposure to light or heat)
- Improper dilutions
- Chemical denaturation
- Contamination
- Adsorption

Factors Related to the Method of Administration
- Injection of too little antigen
- Delayed administration after drawing into syringe
- Injection too deep

Factors Related to Reading the Test and Recording Results
- Inexperienced reader
- Conscious or unconscious bias
- Error in recording

From American Thoracic Society: Diagnostic standards and classification of tuberculosis. Am Rev Respir Dis 142:725–735, 1990.

contraindication for testing.[33] Excluding HIV-positive patients or those with AIDS, only a small proportion of infected people with one of the conditions listed in Table 1 may have a falsely nonsignificant reaction to the test (*see* Table 1). A negative test does not exclude the diagnosis of tuberculosis from further consideration, especially if the person's symptoms are consistent with tuberculosis.

The CDC recommends that any person with HIV infection or believed to be at risk for HIV infection be evaluated for anergy in conduction with PPD testing, with two companion antigens to measure delayed hypersensitivity reactions, such as *Candida* antigen, mumps, or tetanus toxoid.[25,53] A reaction to any of the skin test antigens (including PPD) of 2 mm induration or more signifies that the patient is not anergic; no reaction classifies the patient as anergic.[25] The CDC does not recommend the use of "second strength" antigen (250 TU) for anergy testing.[16]

Interpretation of Test Results

The classification of a tuberculosis skin test reaction as significant or positive is influenced by several factors. Ideally, the definition of a significant test should allow for a clear separation between a reaction due to infection with *M. tuberculosis* and a reaction due to other mycobacterial infections, since there is cross-reactivity between these organisms in skin testing. Using a low cutoff point to demarcate a positive reaction can lead to a large number of false positive results in areas with a high nontuberculous mycobacteria rate or in communities with a low prevalence of tuberculosis infection. Thus, it is important to know the underlying prevalence of tuberculosis in the particular community in which the skin testing occurs. The underlying characteristics of the group tested are of interest: If a population is known to have no exposure to atypical mycobacteria, the specificity of an intermediate strength tuberculosis test, 5 TU, considered positive at 10 mm induration, is essentially 100%.[63] Reactions to these mycobacteria other than tuberculosis, however, tend to have a smaller margin of induration.

The use of a cutoff point of 5 mm to separate significant from nonsignificant reactions prevents very few people from being classified as negative when they are infected with tuberculosis. However, there are many areas, such as the southern United States, in which this cutoff point will lead to the classification of persons as being skin-test positive because they are having a cross-reaction to a mycobacterium other than tuberculosis.

Using a cutoff point based on the person's risk provides the greatest certainty that the result obtained is accurate. For the highest risk groups, a low cutoff of 5 mm is used. People in the highest risk group include HIV-infected persons, recent close contacts of an infected individual (with close contact denoting household exposure or unprotected occupational exposure similar to that of a household exposure, such as in a closed environment) and people with abnormal chest radiographs with fibrotic lesions consistent with old tuberculosis.[12,25]

A higher cutoff, 10 mm, is used for people who are at increased risk for developing tuberculosis but are not in the highest risk group. This includes people with certain medical conditions known to increase the risk of tuberculosis (Table 2); intravenous drug users who are known to be HIV-negative; foreign-born people from countries with a high tuberculosis prevalence; medically underserved people, low-income populations, homeless people; and residents of correctional facilities, nursing homes, and mental institutions. An even higher cutoff is used for all other people with none of these risk factors, since there is a low probability of exposure to tuberculosis and cross-reactivity is more likely to be more common than a

TABLE 2. Medical Conditions That Increase the Risk of Developing Active Tuberculosis, If Infected

Silicosis	Postgastrectomy state
Diabetes mellitus	Peptic ulcer disease
Prolonged steroid use	Chronic malabsorption syndrome
Other immunosuppressive therapy	Post-intestinal bypass
Leukemia	Cancer of the oropharynx or upper gastrointestinal tract
Hodgkin's disease	HIV infection
End-stage renal disease	Abnormal chest x-ray with fibrotic lesions
Rapid weight loss or chronic undernutrition	

From Centers for Disease Control: Core Curriculum on Tuberculosis. Atlanta, Centers for Disease Control, 1991.

reaction caused by tuberculosis infection.[3,12,25] This cutoff of a skin test reaction of ≥ 15 mm was chosen to prevent misclassification of false positive results and as a means of minimizing the use of potentially inappropriate preventive therapy.[5]

People with recent skin-test conversions are considered a high-risk group, because this indicates recently occurring infection. Some authors define a conversion as an increase of at least 6 mm in induration over 2 years, from a reaction of less than 10 mm in diameter on the first test to 10 mm or more on the second test.[7] The CDC has recently defined a conversion as an increase in induration of ≥ 10 mm from a previous skin test within 2 years in people younger than 35 and an induration of ≥ 15 mm in people older than 35.[3] See Table 3 for a summary of the interpretation of skin test results.

The Booster Phenomenon

The booster phenomenon has been reported for more than 50 years. It has been well established that the cutaneous reaction to tuberculin may wane over time, resulting in an apparently negative test in people actually infected with tuberculosis. However, when retested, people show an increase in the size of skin reaction, because their sensitivity to tuberculin is recalled, or boosted.[39,73] Boosting is interpreted as representing waning, preexisting mycobacterial sensitivity that is restored by the antigenic challenge of the initial test.[7] The second test may elicit a significant reaction after an interval as short as a week and as long as a year following the first test.[3,7] A boosted reaction is defined as an increase of at least 6 mm from an original test < 10 mm to a reaction ≥ 10 mm.[65] The booster phenomenon is much more common among elderly people.

In a study of elderly nursing home residents, Stead and To found that boosted reactions reflecting prior tuberculous infection were smaller (< 12 mm increase in size versus the first test) than reactions indicating a recent infection or conversion.[70] Gordin et al. studied a group of chronic care patients for the stability of boosted reactions. Their results indicate that some boosted reactions, especially those < 15 mm of induration, are unstable and may not represent true positive tests.[39] They believe that it is likely that people in whom the positive reaction reverts to negative within 1 year are in fact immunologically incapable of preventing a new infection if exposed to *M. tuberculosis* and should be managed as if they were tuberculin negative.

Accounts of hospital employee screening programs for tuberculosis have shown a common problem: During the early years after institution of surveillance the annual incidence of positive skin-test reactions has been disproportionately high versus the baseline prevalence of positive reactions. This increase seems to

TABLE 3. Summary of Interpretation of Skin Tests

1. A reaction of ≥ 5 mm is classified as positive in
   - people with HIV infection or risk factors for HIV infection with unknown HIV status
   - people who have had recent close contact with persons with active TB*
   - people who have abnormal chest radiographs consistent with old healed TB
2. A reaction of ≥ 10 mm is classified as positive in all people who do not meet any of the criteria above but who have other risk factors for TB including

   High-Risk Groups
   - intravenous drug users known to be HIV seronegative
   - people with other medical conditions that have been reported to increase the risk of progressing from latent TB infection to active TB, including silicosis, gastrectomy, jejuno-ileal bypass surgery, being 10% or more below ideal body weight, chronic renal failure, diabetes mellitus, high-dose corticosteroid and other immunosuppressive therapy, some hematologic disorders (leukemias, lymphomas), and other malignancies

   High-Prevalence Groups
   - foreign-born people from countries in Asia, Africa and Latin America with a high prevalence
   - people from medically underserved low income populations
   - residents of long-term care facilities (correctional institutions, nursing homes)
   - people from high-risk populations in their communities, as determined by local public health authorities
3. Induration of ≥ 15 mm is classified as positive for people who do not meet any of the above criteria.
4. Recent converters are defined on the basis of both induration and age:
   - ≥ 10 mm increase within 2 years is classified as positive for people younger than 35
   - > 15 mm increase within 2 years is classified as positive for people 35 or older
   - ≥ 5 mm increase under circumstances described in #1, above

* Recent close contact implies household contact or unprotected occupations exposure similar in intensity and duration to household contact.

From Centers for Disease Control and Prevention: Draft guidelines for preventing the transmission of tuberculosis in health care facilities, 2nd ed; Notice of comment period. Federal Register 58:52810–52854, October 12, 1993.

occur in the absence of any unusual amounts of exposure to infectous tuberculosis in the hospital.[73] Thompson et al. studied employees at 10 hospitals throughout the United States to address the problem of interpretation of serial testing in hospital employees. Boosted reactions were thought to be more often due to recalled sensitivity to nontuberculous mycobacteria. The conversion rate on subsequent skin tests for the group that was not given an interim test (one within a short interval after the first negative test) was twice the rate found in the group given a second tuberculin test 1 week after the first.[73] Bass et al. found that performing a two-step initial testing procedure for new employees decreased the yearly conversion rate from 8.7% to 2.9% in 1 year. The two-step testing eliminated the age dependency of conversion; there had been a much higher rate of positive reactions in employees older than 50, which was found to be due to boosted reactions. The boosted reaction rate in their workers older than 50 years was 9%.[4]

Sensitization to mycobacteria other than tuberculosis appears to be more subject to boosting than *M. tuberculosis,* which may pose a problem if a screening program takes place in an area with a high prevalence of nontuberculous mycobacteria.[65] In addition, boosted reactions may account for a significant number of "positive" reactions in some groups: A study of Indochinese refugees showed that 52% of people with an initially negative test had a positive result when retested 1–3 weeks later.[54]

Two-step testing procedures can eliminate some difficulties in the proper interpretation of a positive test. The American Thoracic Society and the CDC

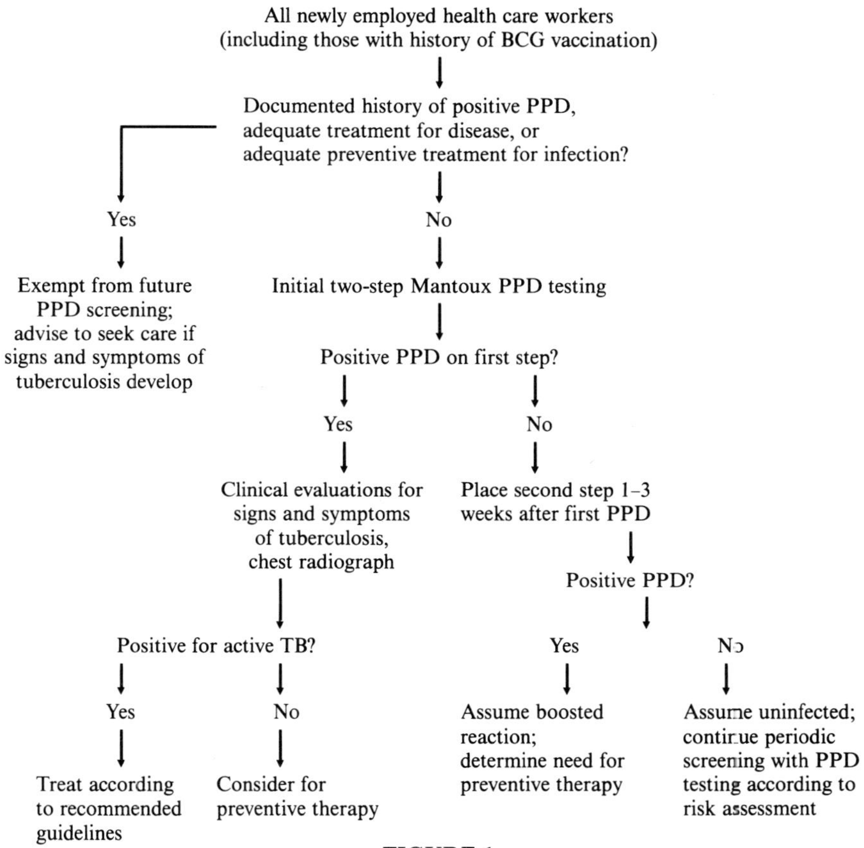

FIGURE 1.

recommend that two-step testing be done on all newly employed health care workers who have an initial negative PPD at the time of employment (Fig. 1).[13,25,33] A second test should be performed 1–3 weeks later. If the second test is positive, this is most likely a boosted reaction, and the person should be classified as previously infected. If the second test remains negative, the person is classified as uninfected. A positive reaction at any time in the future is likely to represent new infection with *M. tuberculosis.*[25] The extra visits to an employee health service generated by the two-step procedure and the cost and discomfort of a second test are a small price to pay for the additional proportion of true tuberculin reactors found and false converters avoided.[65]

The Importance of Bacille Calmette-Guérin (BCG) Vaccination on Skin-Test Results

The BCG vaccine, first used in humans in 1921, was derived from a strain of *Mycobacterium bovis* attenuated through years of serial passage in culture by Calmette and Guérin. The many vaccines available worldwide all have been derived from the original strain, but they vary in culture characteristics and in their ability to induce sensitization to tuberculin.[8] Estimated overall efficacies of the vaccine in preventing infection vary widely. A follow-up study of more than 54,000 participants in England vaccinated with BCG and vole bacillus vaccines found an average 77% efficacy in preventing tuberculosis over 20 years.[42] A Norwegian study estimated the protective effect of BCG to be 80% in the first 10 years after vaccination.[74] A recent meta-analysis quantifying the efficacy of BCG vaccine against tuberculosis compared 14 prospective trials and 12 case-control studies and concluded that BCG vaccine signficantly reduces the risk of tuberculosis by 50%.[31]

The BCG vaccine causes a skin-test reaction that is indistinguishable from a reaction seen after infection with *M. tuberculosis.* The size of the skin test reaction caused by BCG varies by the strain and dose of vaccine used, the age and nutritional status at vaccination, and the frequency of tuberculin testing.[8,67] The persistence of tuberculin sensitivity during the months and years following BCG vaccination is also highly variable. In general, BCG effectiveness wanes over time so that the longer the time from vaccination, the less likely the reaction is due to the vaccine; after 15 years the protective effect is not likely to occur.[67]

Large skin reactions to 5 TU of tuberculin should be considered indicative of infection with *M. tuberculosis,* especially among people from countries with a high prevalence of tuberculosis infection. The mean skin reaction size from BCG vaccination is often < 10 mm.[3] Enhanced reactivity to repeated tuberculin testing is seen in people with prior BCG immunization who have an initial negative reaction to skin testing. Sepulveda observed that positive tuberculin reactions can be present in healthy young adults after BCG administration and that the booster effect of tuberculin testing increases the number of healthy people documented to be tuberculin-positive.[64] Employees with a history of BCG vaccination should undergo skin testing, but it is important for two-step testing to be done to eliminate misclassification of individuals as positive or converters when the reaction is actually due to the booster phenomenon. The same guidelines apply for classification of a skin-test reaction from BCG as a boosted reaction (an increase in reaction size of ≥ 6 mm from a first test reaction of < 10 mm to a test reaction of > 10 mm).

EVALUATION AND MANAGEMENT OF A POSITIVE SKIN TEST

The evaluation and management of a worker with a positive skin test is an integral component of tuberculosis surveillance. The evaluation will determine the extent of treatment required. The use of preventive therapy to prevent both active disease in the worker and the potential for further spread of tuberculosis must be considered. Work restrictions on the infected worker must be based on clearly outlined policies aimed at preventing spread of tuberculosis and ensuring the health and confidentiality of the individual worker. Problem evaluation of the work environment to determine how and why the worker was exposed, and the extent to which others were exposed, is crucial in preventing further transmission of tuberculosis and for eliminating tuberculosis as a workplace hazard.

Evaluation of Health Care Personnel with Positive Skin-Test Reactions

Anyone with a positive skin-test reaction on repeat testing or after exposure to tuberculosis should have a clinical evaluation for the presence of active tuberculosis, including a chest radiograph. If a diagnosis of active tuberculosis is made, appropriate therapy should be instituted.

Personnel with positive skin-test reactions or recent skin test conversions should be evaluated for the use of preventive therapy (see below). Routine chest x-rays are not required for asymptomatic, tuberculosis skin-test–negative health care workers. After the initial chest x-ray is taken in an individual with a positive skin test reaction, it is not necessary to repeat the x-ray unless symptoms suggestive of tuberculosis develop.[25]

If skin test conversions are identified, co-workers from the same work area should be skin-tested to determine if there is additional tuberculosis transmission in the workplace. This is also important for workers who are not regularly assigned to one specific area; efforts should be made to determine the location where they may have been exposed to active tuberculosis.[25] Skin testing should be repeated every 3 months in an area where there has been documented exposure and skin-test conversion, until no additional conversions have occurred for 2 consecutive 3-month periods.[25] The frequency of skin testing should be determined from the risk assessment (see below).

Preventive Therapy for Tuberculosis

Preventive therapy for tuberculosis infection can be used for different purposes: to prevent latent (asymptomatic) infection from progressing to clinical disease, to prevent initial infection, and to prevent recurrence of past, untreated disease.[11] In the United States, there are an estimated 10–15 million asymptomatically infected individuals; more than 90% of current tuberculosis cases arise from this pool. Preventive therapy presumably acts by diminishing the bacterial population in "healed" or radiographically invisible lesions. The beneficial effect of preventive medication in people with a significant tuberculosis skin-test reaction persists for up to 20 years and presumably for life.[1] The proper use of preventive therapies can greatly reduce the incidence of infectious tuberculosis.

Preventive therapy is initiated on less than 60% of infected contacts of people with newly diagnosed tuberculosis.[11] Although 75% of people with newly diagnosed cases of tuberculosis have had contact with a physician in the 5 years prior to diagnosis, less than one third of them have undergone skin testing despite having risk factors for tuberculosis. Glassroth et al. studied people with a positive PPD and other factors placing them at high risk of disease and found that only 5% had been offered preventive therapy.[38] He concluded that there were three main reasons for the failure of preventive therapy: Some patients only have access to health care when they develop active infection; screening and preventive therapy for tuberculosis are not offered; or screening, if performed, may be ineffective at the time of application because a false negative result is obtained.

High-Risk Groups

Certain groups within the TB-infected population are considered to be at high risk for the development of active tuberculosis and should receive the highest priority for preventive therapy. According to the CDC, people with any of the following risk factors should be considered as candidates for preventive therapy, regardless of their age, if they have not had prior treatment:[11]

- Individuals who are HIV-positive or have HIV risk factors if their status is unknown (skin test reaction $\geq$ 5 mm induration)
- Close contacts of people with newly diagnosed infectious tuberculosis ($\geq$5 mm); close contacts are defined as immediate family members, close social contacts, and others (hospital roommates, some health care providers) who share the same indoor environment with an infectious tuberculosis patient for substantial period[20]

- People with abnormal chest x-rays, showing fibrotic lesions likely to represent old healed tuberculosis (≥ 5 mm)
- People with medical conditions that are reported to increase the risk of developing active tuberculosis (≥ 10 mm)
- Recent skin test converters (≥ 10 mm increase within 2 years in people younger than 35; ≥ 15 mm increase for people older than 35)
- Intravenous drug users known to be HIV-seronegative (≥ 10 mm)

In the absence of any of these risk factors, people younger than 35 with ≥10 mm induration from a skin test who belong to the following high-incidence groups are candidates for preventive therapy:[11]

- Foreign born people from countries with a high prevalence
- Medically underserved low-income populations, including high-risk racial or ethnic minority populations, especially black Americans, Hispanics, and Native Americans
- Residents of facilities for long-term care (correctional institutions, nursing homes, and mental institutions)

Staff members of facilities in which an infected individual with active disease would pose a risk to a large number of susceptible people, such as a health care facility, correctional facility, or school or child care facility, should also be considered for preventive therapy if their tuberculin reaction is ≥ 10 mm induration. Health care workers with a positive PPD who do not have any risk factors that increase the likelihood of developing active disease should be considered for preventive therapy if they are younger than 35.[25]

Treatment for Individuals with Positive Tuberculin Skin Tests

Before preventive therapy is given to an individual with a positive skin reaction, the presence of bacteriologically positive or radiologically progressive tuberculosis must be excluded. Every person with a significant tuberculin skin test reaction should have a chest x-ray to rule out active tuberculosis, because active disease requires treatment with multiple antituberculous medications. Individuals should also be questioned to determine whether they have ever received preventive therapy for a positive skin reaction. If so, they would not require any further treatment unless they develop signs and symptoms consistent with tuberculosis.

Isoniazid (INH) is the only medication that has been shown to be effective for preventing active tuberculosis. INH reduces the risk of developing tuberculosis overall by about 70%.[15] If patients take a full regimen, the effectiveness increases to about 93%.[45] A study of infected children in Houston treated with INH demonstrated that the drug was effective 98% of the time.[44] Similar high rates of efficacy were seen in compliant nursing home patients.[71] Problems with compliance arise, in part, due to the long duration of treatment required for adequate protection.

INH is relatively safe, but there are well-known side effects. The most serious is INH-associated hepatic injury. Other side effects, including headaches, nausea, and dizziness, are mild and usually transient.[45] A study of INH use for preventive therapy in the elderly found that nausea, anxiety, somnolence, fever, and skin rash occurred more frequently (8.7%) than hepatitis (1.4%).[37,71] Peripheral neuropathy has been associated with INH but is uncommon at a dose of 5 mg/kg/day. Individuals with other conditions in which neuropathy is common (diabetes, alcoholism, uremia, malnutrition) should receive pyridoxine (vitamin B_6) with the INH.[1] Pyridoxine should also be used in conjunction with INH in pregnant women and in patients with seizure disorders.

INH is normally used alone in preventive therapy at a daily dose of 10 mg/kg, up to a maximum adult dose of 300 mg per day. It can also be given twice a week in a dose of 15 mg/kg, up to 900 mg per dose. INH should be given for a total of 6 months to infected individuals. Patients also infected with HIV, or patients with abnormal chest x-ray consistent with past tuberculosis infection, should receive 12 months of therapy.[11,15] INH was found to have an efficacy of 87% in preventing disease in a Zambian study of patients with both HIV and TB.[76] Rifampin (600 mg/day) for 12 months can be used for preventive therapy for close contacts of individuals with INH-resistant organisms susceptible to rifampin.[15] Although INH does not appear to harm the fetus, preventive therapy should be delayed until after delivery unless the pregnant women has been recently infected. In that instance, INH should be initiated after the infection is documented, but only after the first trimester.[1]

Isoniazid-Associated Hepatitis

Ferebee and Mont demonstrated long-term reductions in tuberculosis morbidity following a year of INH prophylactic treatment in 1962, but a serious risk of liver injury soon became apparent.[46] A large study (13,838 people nationwide) was undertaken by the United States Public Health Service in the 1970s to determine the incidence of INH-related hepatitis. Overall rates of probable and possible cases of hepatitis presumed to be INH-associated (presumed because INH-related toxicity does not cause any pathognomonic liver changes) were 1.3%, with a case fatality rate of 4.6%.[51] The greatest proportion of hepatitis cases occurred in the early months of treatment. Age appeared to be the predominant factor influencing the development of hepatitis: Increasing age was associated with increasing risk, up to age 64.[51] Drinking alcohol, especially on a daily basis, also seemed to enhance the risk of hepatitis among people concurrently taking INH.

While deaths associated with INH-associated hepatitis are probably less frequent than they were in the 1970s, they still occur. A survey of available literature from 1969–1989 found that 69% of INH-related deaths were in women; a high percentage were in women within a year of being postpartum.[68] From 1991–1993, the New York State Department of Health received reports of 10 patients with severe INH-associated liver damage; some required liver transplantation.[23] The median duration of use was 57 days, and seven patients continued to take INH for at least 10 days after the onset of hepatitis symptoms. There have also been reports of severe hepatotoxicity in patients taking INH and ingesting acetominophen.[55]

Benefit-Risk Consideration for the Use of Preventive Therapy

The current recommendations for INH use from the American Thoracic Society include the avoidance of INH preventive therapy in a large proportion of the infected population: people older than 35 with no other risk factors for activation. The age of 35 was chosen as a cutoff for two reasons. Tuberculosis reactivation rates plateau in young adulthood and subsequently decline, and INH-related hepatitis rates increase with age. Since INH prophylaxis was calculated to prevent more cases of tuberculosis than cause cases of hepatitis in people younger than 35, this age limit was incorporated into the American Thoracic Society's recommendations.[32] However, a study of INH use in recent converters in a nursing home found that the incidence of toxicity from the medication was small in the elderly and protected the residents from progression to active disease in 85% of infected individuals.[71]

Even with the age limitations, some authors do not advocate INH preventive therapy. Taylor et al. argue that INH therapy would cause more cases of hepatitis than prevent active tuberculosis.[72] They estimate that treating 100,000 people for 1 year with INH would decrease the number of deaths from tuberculosis during the subsequent 20 years from 33 to 2, but would cause up to 51 deaths due to INH-associated hepatotoxicity during the year of treatment. Israel et al. feel that the current guidelines encouraging the wide use of preventive therapy are unwise, because they inflict a risk of fatal hepatitis on compliant, conscientious adults and older children who have little danger of developing tuberculosis, while those who would benefit more from INH, such as alcohol and drug addicted individuals, are unlikely to comply with a full course of INH therapy.[46]

Rose et al. performed a decision analysis to determine whether preventive therapy with INH was cost-effective in all age groups.[60] They found that INH use in young, high-risk infected people was effective and reduced medical care expenditures. For older, low-risk tuberculin skin test reactors, the benefit of INH was real, but small. However, because the cost of the medications is small, the cost-effectiveness ratio was found to be similar to accepted preventive measures such as the treatments of high cholesterol and hypertension. In another study, Rose et al. found that INH chemoprophylaxis would slightly increase the expected survival and concluded that INH preventive therapy benefits all low-risk tuberculin reactors from age 10–80.[59]

Many of the decision analyses compare tuberculosis cases that were prevented as a result of prophylactic medication with cases of INH-associated hepatitis. However, in addition to the effect on the individual person, halting the progression to active disease prevents the infection of others. In nursing homes, for example, one infected person can spread infection to a large number of the fellow residents, personnel, and visitors.[71]

Some authors advocate the use of BCG vaccination as a strategy to prevent transmission of tuberculosis in the health care setting,[40] especially in light of the low compliance rates seen in some health care workers with tuberculosis screening and INH use. They argue that at current compliance rates, BCG affords greater levels of protection against active tuberculosis than the current strategy of screening followed by INH chemoprevention. However, the American Thoracic Society and CDC do not currently recommend BCG vaccination for health care workers.

Monitoring Procedures for Individuals on Preventive Therapy

Prior to initiating preventive therapy, active tuberculous disease must be excluded. Previous completion of a course of preventive therapy should be ruled out. Specific contraindications to INH use include previous INH-associated hepatic injury, a history of a severe adverse reaction to INH, such as a drug fever or rash, and acute or active liver disease of any cause. Special precautions should be taken in monitoring individuals who are taking INH and who have any of the following factors: concurrent use of any other medication on a long-term basis, alcohol abuse, a history of previous discontinuation of INH due to side effects, chronic liver disease, peripheral neuropathy, pregnancy, postpartum state, or age over 35.[1,15] A transaminase test (ALT or AST) should be performed prior to the onset of INH therapy and periodically during therapy. Routine liver function tests are not recommended for people younger than 35 taking INH, either prior to or during INH treatment unless there are signs and symptoms of toxicity.

If any of these tests exceeds three to five times the laboratory normal, the decision to continue INH therapy must be reconsidered.[1] Approximately 10–20% of individuals receiving INH will develop some mild abnormalities of liver function tests, which tend to resolve even if INH is continued. A positive hepatitis B surface antigen result is not a contraindication for INH use unless it is associated with chronic active hepatitis.[1]

All patients should be monitored at monthly intervals, preferably in person by a health care professional, and educated about the symptoms of hepatitis, including unexplained weight loss, anorexia, nausea, vomiting, fatigue or weakness lasting longer than 3 days, dark urine, icterus, rash, persistent paresthesias of the hands and feet, unexplained elevated temperature for longer than 3 days, and abdominal tenderness, especially in the right upper quadrant.[1] If any of these symptoms are present, individuals should be told to seek medical care immediately and to stop using INH. Liver function tests should be performed in any patient with signs and symptoms of an adverse reaction to INH.

No more than a 1-month supply of isoniazid should be dispensed to the patient at any one time. The careful screening of patients on INH therapy is at present the best way to prevent serious adverse effects in an effort to limit the spread of tuberculosis.

Work Restrictions

Health care workers with active pulmonary and laryngeal tuberculosis can transmit tuberculosis, pose a risk to patients and other health care workers, and should be excluded from work until they are no longer infectious. These work restrictions are universal and do not differ based on the immune status of the worker. Before employees can return to work, the health care facility needs to ensure that they are receiving adequate therapy, that their cough has resolved, and that three consecutive daily sputum smears are negative.[25] Health care facility staff must ensure that the infected health care workers continue with the appropriate antituberculosis therapy for the proper duration and that sputum smears remain negative. Workers with active tuberculosis who discontinue therapy before an adequate course of medication has been completed should be excluded from work until treatment is resumed and an adequate response to therapy is documented, including three consecutive negative sputum smears. Workers with tuberculosis at sites other than the lung or larynx usually do not need to be excluded from work if concurrent pulmonary disease has been ruled out.[25]

Health care workers receiving preventive therapy for latent tuberculosis infection should be allowed to continue with regular work duties; they do not pose a risk to patients or to coworkers.[25] Health care workers with latent infection who cannot take or do not accept or complete a full course of preventive therapy do not need to be excluded from work. They should, however, be counseled about the risks associated with active tuberculosis and should be instructed to seek prompt medical attention for any symptoms that may be due to tuberculosis, especially if they have exposure to high-risk patients or are at high risk of developing active disease themselves.

Problem Evaluation

Once a skin-test conversion has occurred in a health care worker, further investigation should be undertaken to determine the source of exposure for

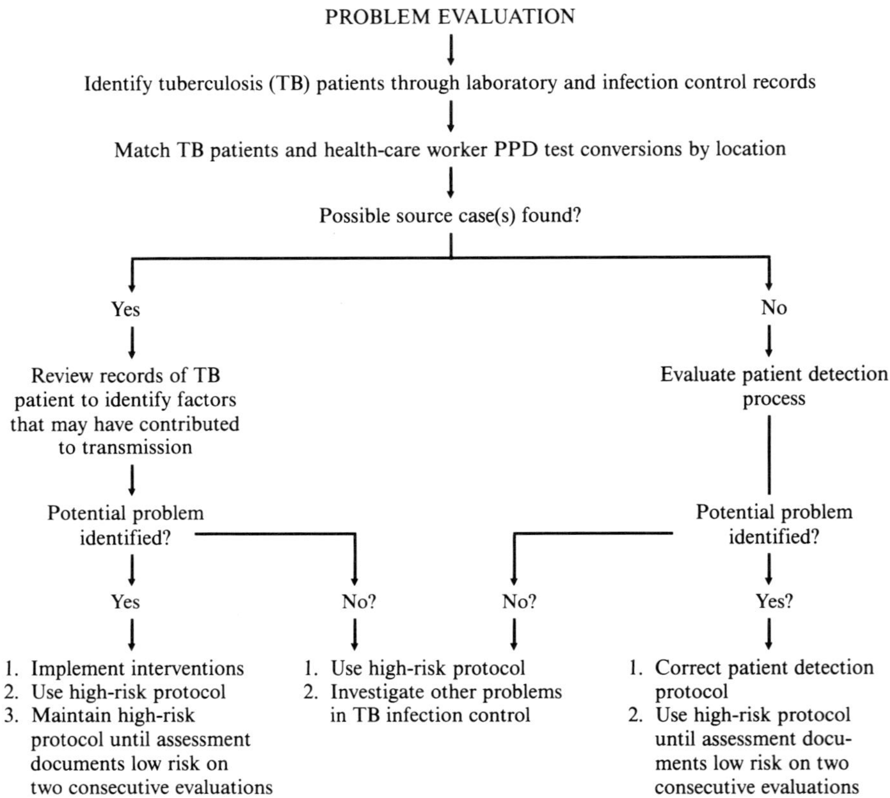

From Centers for Disease Control and Prevention: Draft guidelines for preventing the transmission of tuberculosis in health care facilities, 2nd ed; Notice of comment period. Federal Register 58:52810–52854, October 12, 1993.

FIGURE 2.

remediation and whether other individuals have been similarly exposed and have had skin-test conversions. Figure 2, taken from the CDC's 1993 draft guidelines for preventing transmission of tuberculosis in health care settings, presents a basic algorithm. The CDC outlines the following steps:[25]

1. Prompt evaluation of the health care worker should be performed for evidence of active tuberculosis, including a thorough history, physical examination and chest x-ray.
2. The health care worker should be placed on preventive or curative therapy, whichever is appropriate according to current guidelines.
3. A history of possible exposures should be gathered to try to determine the potential source of tuberculosis infection; once a source of exposure is known, drug susceptibility should be performed on the *M. tuberculosis* isolate to determine the proper preventive therapy.
4. PPD skin testing should be performed on other workers in the area with similar exposure to determine if there is evidence of further transmission. If indicated, contact investigation should be extended to exposed patients.

5. Initiate a problem evaluation, if indicated, with attention to identifying specific problems areas and breakdowns in infection control procedures.

6. If a problem with early TB detection, tuberculosis isolation practices, or engineering controls is identified, appropriate interventions should be implemented. The high-risk protocol (see Risk Assessment) should be followed until there have been two consecutive 3-month periods with no evidence of transmission.

7. If no specific problem can be identified, or the problem does not resolve after the apparent cause has been corrected and no other cause is identified, the high-risk protocol should remain in place in that area, and the public health department or people with expertise in tuberculosis control should be consulted.

When a health care worker develops active tuberculosis, a contact investigation should be performed, including other health care workers and patients and visitors who have had significant exposure to the health care worker. The public health department should be notified both for consultation and to facilitate community contacts not associated with the work environment.

The public health department should notify facilities that a health care worker has developed tuberculosis so that an appropriate contact investigation can be performed at the workplace. The sharing of this information must be strictly limited to protect the confidentiality of the health care worker.

When diagnosis and treatment of a patient with tuberculosis have been delayed, contacts of such patients should be investigated and the following steps taken:[25]

1. Identify health care workers and other patients who were potentially exposed to the tuberculosis patient by interviewing the patients and personnel and reviewing the patient's medical record. The contact investigation should proceed in a concentric circle, expanding from closest to less close contacts, if transmission to the closest contacts is detected.

2. A PPD skin test should be administered to all health care workers and patients with documented exposure as soon as possible after exposure. If the initial test is negative, a repeat test should be administered 12 weeks after the exposure ceased.

3. Exposed persons with skin-test conversions or symptoms suggestive of tuberculosis should be evaluated clinically, including a chest x-ray. People with a history of a positive skin test who have been exposed to an infectious patient do not need a repeat skin test or chest x-ray unless they have symptoms suggestive of tuberculosis.

MULTIDRUG-RESISTANT TUBERCULOSIS

The emergence of multidrug-resistant tuberculosis has caused great concern. In New York City in 1991, 33% of tuberculosis cases were resistant to at least one drug, and 19% of cases were resistant to both isoniazid and rifampin.[22] During 1990–1992, four outbreaks of multidrug-resistant tuberculosis were documented to have occurred, involving nearly 200 cases.[20] The transmission involved patients and health care workers in hospitals and outpatient clinics. Most people with multidrug-resistant tuberculosis in these outbreaks were also infected with HIV. The fatality rate for active multidrug-resistant tuberculosis in individuals who are HIV-positive is 72–89%.[22] Eight health care workers from hospitals with documented outbreaks of multidrug-resistant tuberculosis developed active tuberculosis; four known to be HIV-positive died.[20] All hospital personnel, including volunteers, who may be exposed to patients with expected or known tuberculosis should be educated about the medical consequences of becoming infected with multidrug-resistant tuberculosis and should follow appropriate precautions.[17]

Drug-resistant tubercle bacilli are transmitted in the same manner and with the same likelihood as drug-susceptible organisms. However, people with multidrug-resistant organisms may remain infectious longer and are capable of spreading the disease if they are not on effective therapy.

Factors to consider in the management of people exposed to multidrug-resistant tuberculosis include the likelihood that the contact is newly infected with tuberculosis, the likelihood that the infecting strain is multidrug-resistant, and the estimated likelihood that the contact, if infected, will develop active tuberculosis. High-risk contacts include immediate family members, close social contacts, and others who shared the same indoor environment with an infectious tuberculosis patient for substantial periods.[20] This can also apply to occupational contacts. Individuals without a history of a positive skin test should undergo PPD testing and, if indicated, a chest x-ray and sputum examination. A skin-test reaction of ≥ 5 mm should be considered to indicate new infection, and individuals should be evaluated for preventive therapy after active tuberculosis has been ruled out. Contacts not known or likely to be immunosuppressed with a previously documented positive skin test is probably not newly infected and needs no further evaluation unless symptoms of tuberculosis are present. They should be evaluated for preventive therapy on the basis of the prior positive skin test.

High-risk contacts with an initially negative skin test should receive a follow-up skin test 12 weeks after exposure to tuberculosis has ended. People who initially test negative should be considered newly infected, receive a screening chest x-ray, and be considered for preventive therapy until follow-up testing is negative if there is evidence of tuberculosis contagion among other similarly exposed contacts, or if the contact is a child, HIV-infected (especially if they are known to be anergic), or immunosuppressed. Once the 12-week follow-up skin test is negative, preventive therapy can be safely stopped.[20]

After it has been determined that contacts are newly infected and were exposed to patients with multidrug-resistant tuberculosis, they should be evaluated to assess the likelihood of infection with the multidrug-resistant strain. Considerations should include the infectiousness of the possible source, the closeness and intensity of the exposure, and the contact's likelihood of exposure to people with drug-susceptible tuberculosis.[20] The most important factor determining whether infected individuals will develop active disease is the state of the immune system: Any degree of immunosuppression increases the likelihood, but HIV infection is the greatest factor. Age also plays a role; people younger than 5 and older than 60 have high tuberculosis disease attack rates and shorter incubation periods.

The management of newly infected people varies with the risk of infection with multidrug-resistant tuberculosis. Drug susceptibility tests should be conducted on the tuberculosis isolate of the presumed source(s) to determine the characteristics of the mycobacteria.[17] Individuals believed to have low to low-intermediate likelihood of infection with multidrug-resistant tuberculosis should be managed according to standard recommendations for drug-susceptible tuberculosis patients. People at intermediate to high likelihood of infection with multidrug-resistant tuberculosis need to be subdivided according to risk of developing active disease by level of immunosuppression (known or suspected HIV seropositivity, or other). Preventive therapy for people likely to be infected with multidrug-resistant tuberculosis and at high risk for developing active disease should include at least two drugs. For people not infected with HIV or at risk for HIV infection or otherwise immunosuppressed and who are believed to be infected with a strain 100% resistant to INH and rifampin, two options are available. One option is not to institute immediate preventive therapy and to closely follow them for any indication of active tuberculosis. Alternatively, consideration can be given to multidrug preventive therapy with medications other than INH and rifampin. If resistance to either of these medications is less than 100%, INH and/or rifampin should be used. Possible alternative drug regimens include pyrazinamide and ethambutol, or pyrazinamide plus a fluoroquinolone, such as ofloxacin or ciprofloxacin. Close follow-up of patients on these alternative preventive therapies is indicated, including regular examinations and chest x-rays.[20] The duration of therapy is the same as for drug-susceptible strains: 6 months unless the individual is seropositive for HIV, in which case treatment should last 12 months.

It is currently unknown whether vaccination with BCG vaccines will protect health care workers against tuberculosis, including multidrug-resistant tuberculosis. The vaccines are not recommended by the CDC for use in health care workers and also are contraindicated for use in HIV-infected individuals.[2]

COMPONENTS OF A SCREENING PROGRAM FOR TUBERCULOSIS IN HEALTH CARE WORKERS

Tuberculosis screening and prevention programs should be established in health care settings to protect both the workers and the patients. A comprehensive education program, targeted to the various job categories, should be undertaken as part of the screening program. This training should occur at hiring and periodically thereafter. Table 4 outlines the following elements, which, according to the CDC, should be included in any health care worker education program about tuberculosis.[25]

Counseling the health care worker about tuberculosis is an important component of any comprehensive screening program. Because of increased risk of tuberculosis infection, the CDC recommends that ". . . all HCWs should know if they have a medical condition or are receiving a medical treatment that may lead to severely impaired cell-mediated immunity. HCWs who may be at risk for HIV infection should know their HIV status, i.e., they should be encouraged to voluntarily seek counseling and testing for HIV antibody status. Existing guidelines for counseling and testing should be followed."[25] This knowledge will allow for the correct interpretation of the worker's PPD test and length of time of any indicated preventive therapy, since guidelines vary depending on the individual's underlying health status. Workers may then consider voluntary work reassignment as a result. Knowledge of immune status is especially important when health care workers are exposed to multidrug-resistant tuberculosis. Ideally, for the best protection, severely immunocompromised workers should avoid any exposure to tuberculosis and should consider a change in job setting if their current assignment places them at risk of exposure. Therefore, as stated by the CDC, "HCWs should be advised of options for severely immunocompromised HCWs to voluntarily transfer to areas and activities in which there is the lowest possible risk of exposure to *M. tuberculosis*. This should be a personal decision for HCWs. . . ."[25]

The CDC guidelines also define the employer's responsibility:[25] "Employers should make reasonable attempts to offer alternative job assignments to an employee with a documented condition compromising cell-mediated immunity who works in a high-risk setting for TB. Immunocompromised HCWs should be referred to an

TABLE 4. Elements of a Tuberculosis Education Program

1. Basic concepts about tuberculosis transmission, pathogenesis, diagnosis, including the difference between active tuberculosis and latent tuberculosis infection, the signs and symptoms of active tuberculosis, and the possibility of re-infection in people with a positive skin test
2. The potential for occupational exposure to people with active tuberculosis in the work environment (the health care facility) and situations with increased risk of exposure to tuberculosis
3. Principles and practices of infection control that reduce the risk of transmission of tuberculosis, including the infection control policy of each institution as a whole and situations within the institution with increased risk of tuberculosis exposure
4. The purpose of tuberculosis skin testing with PPD, the importance of participation in skin testing programs, and the significance of a positive test result
5. Basic tenets of preventive therapy for tuberculosis infection, including indications for use and any potential adverse effects of the medication
6. Importance of the health care worker seeking prompt medical education if symptoms suggestive of tuberculosis develop, or if PPD skin test conversion occurs in order to properly treat and prevent the spread of tuberculosis to patients and other health care workers
7. Principles of drug therapy for active tuberculosis disease
8. Importance of notifying the health care facility if active infection develops so that proper contact investigation can be undertaken to limit the spread of infection
9. Responsibility of the employer to maintain confidentiality of the infected worker and to ensure that the worker receives proper therapy and is no longer infectious prior to returning to work
10. The higher risk posed by tuberculosis to individuals with HIV infection or other causes of impaired cell-mediated immunity, including the more frequent and rapid development of clinical disease after infection, differences in disease presentation in people with immunodeficiency and people with intact immune systems, and higher mortality rates seen after infection of immunosuppressed individuals with multidrug-resistant tuberculosis
11. Potential development of anergy as immunodeficiency progresses, potentially making skin testing less sensitive
12. An explanation of the employer's policy on voluntary work reassignment options for immunocompromised individuals

From Centers for Disease Control and Prevention: Draft guidelines for preventing the transmission of tuberculosis in health care facilities, 2nd ed; Notice of comment period. Federal Register, 58:52810–52854, October 12, 1993.

employee health professional who can counsel the employee on an individual basis regarding his/her risk of TB. Upon the request of the immunocompromised HCW, the facility should offer, but not compel, a work setting in which the HCW would have the lowest possible risk of occupational exposure to *M. tuberculosis*." As with all patient information, it is essential that any information provided to the health care facility by the worker about their immune status be handled confidentially, including requests for voluntary job reassignment. There should be written procedures within the institution for handling these matters confidentially.

Health care workers with a cough lasting longer than 2 weeks, especially if it is accompanied by other signs and symptoms associated with tuberculosis such as weight loss, fatigue, night sweats, anorexia, fevers, or bloody sputum, should be evaluated for active tuberculosis with a clinical evaluation, chest radiograph, and sputum sample. Workers should not return to the workplace until active tuberculosis has been ruled out or they are taking appropriate therapy and rendered noninfectious.[25]

Health care workers should be skin-tested using a Mantoux PPD at the time of employment, including employees with a history of past BCG vaccination unless they have a history of a documented positive skin test, are known to have completed a course of adequate preventive therapy, or have had adequate, documented therapy for active disease. These workers should be exempt from further tuberculosis screening unless they develop symptoms suggestive of tuberculosis.[25] However, employees with a history of a positive skin test are at risk for contracting tuberculosis in the future and should be advised and reminded periodically that the onset of symptoms suggestive of tuberculosis should be promptly reported.[13]

The initial skin test should follow the previously detailed two-step testing procedure to minimize skin test "conversions" that are actually due to the boosting phenomenon.[13,25,33] Periodic tuberculosis screening should be performed on all health care workers at intervals determined by the risk assessment (see below).

After the test has been administered, read, and interpreted according to current guidelines,[3,25] workers should be informed about the results and significance of the skin testing.

Records of tuberculosis skin-test results should be kept in both the employee's confidential medical record and in a retrievable aggregate database containing the results of all worker skin-testing results.[25] These results should be periodically analyzed as a part of the risk assessment to determine the risk of contracting tuberculosis among workers in the health care facility as a whole.

THE ROLE OF PPD TESTING IN RISK ASSESSMENT

A PPD skin testing program, if carefully conducted and properly analyzed, can provide essential information about the adequacy of TB infection control. Indeed, in the latest draft guidelines from the CDC, issued in December 1993, the results of PPD testing form a central component of the process of determining the level of risk of TB infection in the health care setting, which, in turn, constitutes the basis of an appropriate TB infection control program.[25]

From an occupational health perspective, however, PPD testing, like any workplace-based medical surveillance program, has limitations. On a practical level, instituting and maintaining a rigorous skin testing program with a high rate of compliance is difficult and costly. Employee health services are rarely given the money that they require. On a conceptual level, PPD testing is also defective. By its nature as a measurement of infection, PPD testing relies on the failure of controls in order to yield useful information. PPD testing may help prevent future exposure to *M. tuberculosis* but contributes little prospectively to the primary prevention of infection. In occupational health, a direct assessment of the integrity of environmental and administrative controls has conceptual primacy over medical surveillance, since they limit exposure in the first place.

This section outlines the use of PPD testing in the risk assessment process drafted by the CDC in December 1993.[25] The CDC guidelines are expected to be finalized in late 1994, and the reader is advised to consult with the final version to determine if there are any significant changes from the draft version.

The CDC states that the purpose of risk assessment is "to evaluate the risk of TB transmission in each area and occupational group in the facility so that appropriate infection control interventions can be developed based on actual risk."[25] The risk assessment process needs to be applied to the institution as a whole, to functional areas within the institution such as emergency departments and medicine wards, and to so-called "occupational groups" of workers such as respiratory therapists, doctor aides, maintenance, and other workers whose jobs require that they move throughout the health care facility.

The risk assessment process relies upon two types of data to judge risk: (1) PPD test results and (2) information about TB patients in the health care facility. An increased potential for TB transmission to workers is present if any of the following conditions are met:[25]

1. The PPD conversion rate for a given area or occupational group is higher than the rate in comparable areas or groups with no known contact with TB patients
2. A cluster of PPD conversions occurs, i.e., two or more PPD conversions occur in an area or occupational group within 3 months
3. Six or more patients with TB are treated per year in that area
4. Evidence of patient-to-patient transmission of TB is present

The CDC guidelines do not set any fixed number for how much higher the rate of PPD conversions must be to attain significance as a reflection of risk. Statistical significance testing may be useful, but its overuse is specifically discouraged, especially when small numbers of workers are being tested.

These four empirically derived items are combined to form three categories of risk: low, intermediate, and high. Each area or occupational group is assigned a risk category which is used to determine the frequency of PPD testing, periodic risk assessment, evaluation of the ventilation system, and the need for urgent problem evaluation and the enhancement of engineering and administrative controls.

The criteria and recommended activities for low-, intermediate-, and high-risk categories are illustrated in Table 5, which is modified from the December 1993

TABLE 5. Risk Assessment Criteria and Actions[25]

	Criteria for Determining Risk Category	Risk Category	Actions Based on Risk Category
			Time Interval for: • PPD testing • Risk assessment • Ventilation system testing
1. Is PPD conversion rate in work area greater than previously or greater than in other areas? 2. Is there a cluster of PPD conversions?[1] 3. Is there evidence of patient-to-patient transmission?	No to all 3 criteria → $\leq$6 TB patients in area/year →	Low risk	Every 12 months
	No to all 3 criteria → >6 TB patients in area/year →	Intermediate risk[2]	Every 6 months
	Yes to any of the 3 criteria →	High risk	Every 3 months Additional measures • Initiate problem evaluation • Consider supplemental engineering measures • Maintain high index of suspicion for TB patients

[1] Cluster = Two or more PPD conversions in one area or a single occupational group that works in multiple areas over a 3-month period.

[2] Occurrence of drug-resistant TB in the facility or the community, or high prevalence of HIV infection among patients or workers in the facility may warrant a higher risk rating.

draft CDC guidelines. Low and intermediate risk categories share the absence of an elevated PPD test conversion rate, the absence of a PPD cluster, and the lack of evidence of patient-to-patient transmission. They differ only in two regards. The low-risk category is reserved for areas with fewer than six tuberculosis patients per year, and the intermediate category refers to areas with six or more such patients. The two categories also differ in the frequency of recommended actions: every 12 months for the low-risk category and every 6 months for the intermediate-risk category (*see* Table 5).

The designation of a high-risk category is reserved for areas or groups with one or more items of evidence of increased TB risk: an elevated rate of PPD conversions, a cluster of PPD test conversions, or evidence of TB transmission from patient to patient or patient to worker. In high-risk areas, problem evaluation should be done immediately, followed by the PPD testing, periodic risk assessment, and evaluation of the ventilation system every 3 months. Following problem identification and intervention, the level of risk may be downgraded to the appropriate level when two consecutive 3-month periods show no evidence of further tuberculosis transmission.

Areas of the health care facility where cough-inducing procedures are performed (bronchoscopy, sputum induction, aerosol therapy) are considered intermediate risk unless they meet one of the criteria cited above that would elevate them to the high-risk category. Also, an increase in the risk category should be considered for areas or occupational groups in which drug-resistant tuberculosis occurs with significant frequency or where there is a high prevalence of HIV infection among either patients or workers.[25]

Tuberculosis infection control programs should include periodic skin testing with purified protein derivative and risk assessment of the working environment. An initial risk assessment should be performed to evaluate the risk of tuberculosis transmission in each area and occupational group in the facility to allow appropriate measures to be instituted based on the actual risk.[25] The initial risk assessment should be done for the entire institution as well as areas where tuberculosis patients may be cared for or where high-risk procedures such as cough-producing procedures are performed. Individual groups of health care workers throughout the institution should also be assessed for risk levels. Institutional skin-test conversion records should be kept confidential, and rates should be determined for the various groups and areas of the hospital, using the number of workers in an area or group as the denominator and the number of skin-test conversions within each segment as the numerator.

Health care workers must be skin-tested at the time of employment, including employees with past BCG vaccination, unless a previously positive reaction can be documented, or completion of adequate preventive therapy or adequate therapy for active disease can be documented. Workers with a documented history of a positive skin test or those who have received adequate preventive therapy or appropriate therapy for active tuberculosis should be exempt from further screening unless they develop symptoms that are suggestive of tuberculosis.

REGULATORY REQUIREMENTS FOR PPD TESTING

In 1993, the federal Occupational Safety and Health Administration (OSHA) developed a national enforcement policy and procedures for occupational exposure to tuberculosis. This policy and procedures were based in part upon the experience of OSHA Region II (New York and New Jersey) and the New York

State Department of Health's Public Employee Safety and Health Program in the issuance and enforcement of guidelines in April 1992. Although the federal OSHA policy applies only to the private sector and federal agencies, states with occupational safety and health regulations for public employees usually adopt federal OSHA standards; therefore, it is likely that state and municipal workers have or will be covered by guidelines that are at least as strict as the federal OSHA guidelines. The national OSHA policy does not constitute a specific regulatory standard but relies for its authority principally on its so-called general duty clause (Sec 5(a)(1)) of the Occupational Safety and Health Act of 1970. A full airborne infectious disease standard awaits future action by OSHA.

The medical surveillance provisions of the 1993 OSHA guidelines rely on CDC's 1990 *Guidelines for Preventing the Transmission of Tuberculosis in Health Care Settings, with Special Focus on HIV-related Issues*,[13] which are currently undergoing revision. As stated in the memorandum issuing the 1993 OSHA enforcement policy, OSHA expects that, after the publication of the new CDC guidelines, it will issue a compliance directive that will be based on the new CDC guidelines and that will supersede its enforcement policy issued in October 1993. In this directive, OSHA is likely to alter the medical surveillance provisions described in the October 1993 memorandum. However, until that time, the 1993 OSHA guidelines will be in effect.

In the 1993 guidelines, OSHA defines the type of workplaces that are subject to the guidelines and the elements of a medical surveillance program that must be developed for employees in these workplaces. Workplaces must meet the OSHA guidelines if (a) they are one of the following: health care settings, correctional institutions, homeless shelters, long-term care facilities for the elderly, and drug treatment centers, and if (b) employees have potential exposure to suspected or confirmed cases of tuberculosis or engage in a high-risk procedure on TB patients. Employers in such covered facilities must establish a medical surveillance program that includes testing with the Mantoux skin test, evaluation and management of workers with a positive skin test, and training and information about medical surveillance and therapy along with other topics relevant to TB recognition and control.

PPD skin testing must be performed on a pre-placement basis at the time of employment and on an annual basis to all employees in covered facilities. Workers who meet criterion (b) above must have PPD testing every six months. Workers who experience a TB exposure incident must be treated according to a protocol described above. Workers with a positive skin test, a skin test conversion, or symptoms of TB must have appropriate evaluation and management at no cost to the employees. All records relating to TB exposure, skin testing, evaluation, and treatment must be maintained according to the OSHA medical record standard.[29]

As with any occupational illness, OSHA requires that individuals with positive PPD tests or active tuberculosis be recorded on the employer's OSHA 200 log.[30] Workers with positive PPDs on preplacement testing are not required to be listed on the 200 log. However, workers, presumably already employed, who show positive PPDs on baseline testing must be listed on the 200 log "because there is a presumption of work-relatedness in these settings."

REFERENCES

1. American Thoracic Society: Treatment of tuberculosis and tuberculous infection in adults and children. Am Rev Respir Dis 134:355–363, 1986.

2. American Thoracic Society: Mycobacterioses and the acquired immunodeficiency syndrome. Am Rev Respir Dis 138:492–496, 1987.
3. American Thoracic Society: Diagnostic standards and classification of tuberculosis. Am Rev Respir Dis 142:725–735, 1990.
4. Bass JB, Sanders RV, Kirkpatrick MB: Choosing an appropriate cutting point for conversions in annual tuberculin skin testing. Am Rev Respir Dis 132:379–381, 1985.
5. Bass JB Jr: Tuberculin test, preventive therapy, and elimination of tuberculosis [editorial]. Am Rev Respir Dis 141:812–813, 1990.
6. Bellin E, Fletcher D, Safyer S: Abnormal chest x-rays in intravenous drug users: Implications for tuberculosis screening programs. Am J Public Health 83:698–700, 1993.
7. Cauthen GM, Snider DE Jr: Delayed tuberculin boosting in the older population [editorial]. Am Rev Respir Dis 134:857–858, 1986.
8. Centers for Disease Control: Use of BCG vaccines in the control of tuberculosis: A joint statement by the ACIP and the Advisory Committee for Elimination of Tuberculosis. Recommendations of the Immunization Practices Advisory Committee. MMWR 37:663–675, 1988.
9. Centers for Disease Control: A strategic plan for the elimination of tuberculosis in the United States. MMWR 38(S-3):1–25, 1989.
10. Centers for Disease Control: Prevention and control of tuberculosis in correctional institutions: Recommendations of the Advisory Committee for the Elimination of Tuberculosis. MMWR 38:313–320, 325, 1989.
11. Centers for Disease Control: The use of preventive therapy for tuberculous infection in the United States: Recommendations of the Advisory Committee for the Elimination of Tuberculosis. MMWR 39(RR-8):9–12, 1990.
12. Centers for Disease Control: Prevention and control of tuberculosis in facilities providing long-term care to the elderly: Recommendations of the Advisory Committee for the Elimination of Tuberculosis. MMWR 39(RR-10):7–13, 1990.
13. Centers for Disease Control: Guidelines for preventing the transmission of tuberculosis in health care settings, with special focus on HIV-related issues. MMWR 39(RR-17):1–29, 1990.
14. Centers for Disease Control: Tuberculosis among foreign-born persons entering the United States: Recommendations of the Advisory Committee for the Elimination of Tuberculosis. MMWR 39(RR-18):1–22, 1990.
15. Centers for Disease Control: Core Curriculum on Tuberculosis. Atlanta, Centers for Disease Control, 1991.
16. Centers for Disease Control: Purified protein derivative (PPD)-tuberculin anergy and HIV infection: Guidelines for anergy testing and management of anergic persons at risk of tuberculosis. MMWR 40:27–33, 1991.
17. Centers for Disease Control: Nosocomial transmission of multidrug-resistant tuberculosis among HIV-infected persons—Florida and New York, 1988–1991. MMWR 40:585–591, 1991.
18. Centers for Disease Control: Tuberculosis morbidity in the United States: Final data, 1990. MMWR 40(SS-3):23–27, 1991.
19. Centers for Disease Control: Prevention and control of tuberculosis in U.S. communities with at-risk minority populations: Recommendations of the Advisory Council for the Elimination of Tuberculosis and prevention and control of tuberculosis among homeless persons: Recommendations of the Advisory Council for the Elimination of Tuberculosis. MMWR 41(RR-5):1–11, 1992.
20. Centers for Disease Control: National action plan to combat multidrug-resistant tuberculosis: Meeting the challenge of multidrug-resistant tuberculosis; summary of a conference; management of persons exposed to multidrug-resistant tuberculosis. MMWR 41(RR-11):61–71, 1992.
21. Centers for Disease Control: Control of Tuberculosis in Correctional Facilities: A Guide for Health Care Workers. Atlanta, Centers for Disease Control, 1992.
22. Centers for Disease Control: Initial therapy for tuberculosis in the era of multidrug resistance: Recommendations of the Advisory Council for the Elimination of Tuberculosis. MMWR 42(RR-7)1–8, 1993.
23. Centers for Disease Control: Severe isoniazid associated hepatitis—New York, 1991–1993. MMWR 42:545–547, 1993.
24. Centers for Disease Control: Tuberculosis morbidity—United States, 1992. MMWR 42:696–697, 703–704, 1993.
25. Centers for Disease Control and Prevention: Draft guidelines for preventing the transmission of tuberculosis in health care facilities, 2nd ed, Notice of comment period. Federal Register 58:52810–52854, October 12, 1993.

26. Chaparas SD, Vandiviere HM, Melvin I, et al: Tuberculin test: Variability with the Mantoux procedure. Am Rev Respir Dis 132:175–177, 1985.
27. [Reference deleted.]
28. Clague JE, Fields P, Graham DR, Davies PDO: Screening for tuberculosis: Current practices and attitudes of hospital workers. Tubercle 72:265–267, 1991.
29. Code of Federal Regulations: 29 CFR 1910.20. Access to employee exposure and medical records.
30. Code of Federal Regulation: 29 CFR 1904. Log and summary of occupational injuries and illnesses.
31. Colditz GA, Brewer TF, Berkey CS: et al: Efficacy of BCG vaccine in the prevention of tuberculosis: Meta-analysis of the published literature. JAMA 271:698–702, 1994.
32. Colice GL: Decision analysis, public health policy, and isoniazid chemoprophylaxis for young adult tuberculin skin reactors. Arch Intern Med 150:2517–2522, 1990.
33. Comstock GW, Daniel TM, Snider DE, et al: The tuberculin skin test: A statement by the Committee on Diagnostic Skin Testing. Am Rev Respir Dis 124:356–363, 1981.
34. Comstock GW, Edwards PQ: The competing risks of tuberculosis and hepatitis for adult tuberculin reactors [editorial]. Am Rev Respir Dis 111:573–577, 1975.
35. Cross ER, Hyams KC: Tuberculin skin testing in US Navy and Marine Corps personnel and recruits, 1980–1986. Am J Public Health 80:435–438, 1990.
36. De March-Ayuela P: Choosing an appropriate criterion for true and false conversion in serial tuberculin testing. Am Rev Respir Dis 141:815–820, 1990.
37. Dutt AK, Mooers D, Stead WW: Smear negative, culture positive pulmonary tuberculosis: Six-month chemotherapy with isoniazid and rifampin. Am Rev Respir Dis 141:1232–1235, 1990.
38. Glassroth J, Bailey WC, Hopewell PC, et al: Why tuberculosis is not prevented. Am Rev Respir Dis 141:1236–1240, 1990.
39. Gordin FM, Perez-Stable EJ, Reid M, et al: Stability of positive tuberculin tests: Are boosted reactions valid? Am Rev Respir Dis 141:560–563, 1991.
40. Greenberg PD, Lax KG, Schechter CB: Tuberculosis in house staff: A decision analysis comparing the tuberculin screening strategy with the BCG vaccination. Am Rev Respir Dis 143:490–495, 1991.
41. Hanson CA, Reichman LB: Tuberculosis skin testing and preventive therapy. Semin Respir Infect 4:182–188, 1989.
42. Hart PD, Sutherland I: BCG and vole bacillus vaccines in the prevention of tuberculosis in adolescence and early adult life: Final report to the Medical Research Council. BMJ 2:293–295, 1977.
43. Howard TP, Solomon DA: Reading the tuberculin skin test: Who, when, and how? Arch Intern Med 148:2457–2459, 1988.
44. Hsu KH: Thirty years after isoniazid: Its impact on tuberculosis in children and adolescents. JAMA 251:1283–1285, 1984.
45. International Union Against Tuberculosis Committee on Prophylaxis: Efficacy of various durations of isoniazid preventive therapy for tuberculosis: Five years of follow-up in the IUAT trial. Bull WHO 60:555–564, 1982.
46. Israel HL, Gottlieb JE, Maddrey WC: Perspective: Preventive isoniazid therapy and the liver. Chest 101:1298–1301, 1992.
47. Johnson MP, Coberly JS, Clermon HC, Chaison RE, et al: Tuberculin skin test reactivity among adults infected with human immunodeficiency virus. J Infect Dis 166:194–198, 1992.
48. Joint Tuberculosis Committee: Control and prevention of tuberculosis in Britain: An updated code of practice. BMJ 300:995–999, 1990.
49. Kallay MC, Bell KM, Montalbaon B: False positive reactions to aplisol (Parke-Davis) with serial PPD skin testing. Am Rev Respir Dis 135(suppl):A45, 1987.
50. Kochi A: The global tuberculosis situation and the new control strategy of the World Health Organization. Tubercle 72:1–6, 1991.
51. Koparoff DE, Snider DE, Caras GJ: Isoniazid-related hepatitis: A U.S. Public Health Service cooperative study. Am Rev Respir Dis 117:991–1001, 1978.
52. Malasky C, Jordan T, Potulski F, Reichman LB: Occupational tuberculosis infections among pulmonary physicians in training. Am Rev Respir Dis 142:505–507, 1990.
53. Markowitz N, Hansen NI, Wilcosky TC, et al: Tuberculin and anergy testing in HIV-seropositive and HIV-seronegative persons. Ann Intern Med 119:185–193, 1993.
54. Morse DL, Hansen RE, Grabau JC, et al: Tuberculin conversions in Indochinese refugees: An assessment of boosting and anergy. Am Rev Respir Dis 132:516–519, 1985.
55. Murphy R, Swartz R, Watkins PB: Severe acetominophen toxicity in a patient receiving isoniazid. Ann Intern Med 113:799–800, 1990.

56. Nardell ED: Dodging droplet nuclei: Reducing the probability of nosocomial tuberculosis transmission in the AIDS era [editorial]. Am Rev Respir Dis 142:501–503, 1990.
57. Nash DR, Douglass JE: Anergy in active pulmonary tuberculosis: A comparison between positive and negative reactors and an evaluation of 5TU and 250TU skin test doses. Chest 77:32–37, 1980.
58. New York State Department of Health Public Employees Safety and Health: Enforcement Guidelines for Occupational Exposure to Tuberculosis. Albany, April 1992.
59. Rose DN, Schechter CB, Silver AL: The age threshold for isoniazid chemoprophylaxis: A decision analysis for low-risk tuberculin reactors. JAMA 256:2709–2713, 1986.
60. Rose DN, Schechter CB, Fahs MC, Silver AL: Tuberculous prevention: Cost-effectiveness analysis of isoniazid chemoprophylaxis. Am J Prev Med 4:102–109, 1988.
61. Rudd RM, Gellert AR, Venning M: Comparison of Mantoux, tine, and 'Imotest' tuberculin tests. Lancet 2:515–518, 1982.
62. Sbarbaro JA: Skin testing in the diagnosis of tuberculosis. Semin Respir Infect 1:234–238, 1986.
63. Schechter CB, Rose DN, Fahs MC, Silver AL: Tuberculin screening: Cost-effectiveness analysis of various testing schedules. Am J Prev Med 6:167–175, 1990.
64. Sepulveda RL, Ferrer X, Latrach C, Sorensen RU: The influence of Calmette-Guérin bacillus immunization on the booster effect of tuberculin testing in healthy young adults. Am Rev Respir Dis 142:24–28, 1990.
65. Slutkin G, Perez-Stable EJ, Hopewell PC: Time course and boosting of tuberculin reactions in nursing home residents. Am Rev Respir Dis 134:1048–1051, 1986.
66. Snider DE Jr, Anderson HR, Bentley SE: Current tuberculosis screening practices. Am J Public Health 74:1353–1356, 1984.
67. Snider DE Jr: Bacille Calmette-Guérin vaccination and tuberculin skin tests. JAMA 253:3438–3439, 1985.
68. Snider DE Jr, Caras GJ: Isoniazid-associated hepatitis deaths: A review of available information. Am Rev Respir Dis 145:494–497, 1992.
69. Sokal JE: Measurement of delayed skin-test responses. N Engl J Med 293:501–502, 1975.
70. Stead WW, To T: The significance of the tuberculin skin test in elderly persons. Ann Intern Med 107:837–842, 1987.
71. Stead WW, To T, Harrison RW, Abraham JH III: Benefit risk considerations in preventive treatment for tuberculosis in elderly persons. Ann Intern Med 107:843–845, 1987.
72. Taylor WC, Aronson MD, Delbanco TL: Should young adults with a positive tuberculin test take isoniazid? Ann Intern Med 94:808–813, 1981.
73. Thompson NJ, Glassroth JL, Snider DE Jr, Farer LS: The booster phenomenon in serial tuberculin testing. Am Rev Respir Dis 119:587–597, 1979.
74. Tverdal A, Funnemark E: Protective effect of BCG vaccination in Norway 1956–1973. Tubercle 69:119–123, 1988.
75. US Department of Labor, Occupational Safety and Health Administration: Enforcement guidelines for occupational exposure to tuberculosis. April 1992.
76. Wadhawan D, Hira S, Mwansa N, et al: Preventive tuberculosis chemotherapy with isoniazid among persons infected with human immunodeficiency virus [abstract]. Proceedings of the Seventh International Conference on AIDS, Florence, Italy, June 16–21, 1991.
77. Woolf SH: Analytic principles in assessing the effectiveness of clinical preventive services. In Goldman RB, Lawrence RS (eds): Preventing Disease Beyond the Rhetoric. New York, Springer-Verlag, 1990.

SUSAN KLITZMAN, DrPH
PAMELA KELLNER, RN, MPH

CONTROL OF TUBERCULOSIS IN THE WORKPLACE: TOWARD AN INTEGRATION OF OCCUPATIONAL HEALTH AND PUBLIC HEALTH

From the New York City Department of Health
New York, New York

Reprint requests to:
Susan Klitzman, DrPH
New York City Department of Health
125 Worth Street
Box 34C
New York, NY 10013

The resurgence of tuberculosis poses many new challenges for controlling transmission in the workplace. In this article we examine successful models from the past and new challenges for occupational health and public health. We argue that traditional approaches used in both occupational and public health for controlling and preventing disease are not sufficient to control the current TB epidemic. The need for cooperation between public health and occupational health is more urgent than ever; we examine current efforts at and obstacles to forging the link.

The demographic groups most affected by the current tuberculosis epidemic—the homeless, the immunocompromised, drug users, prisoners, and immigrants from countries where there is a high rate of TB—receive services from an expanding number and variety of occupational groups. Members of these groups have a higher risk of TB, either because they are more likely to have been exposed or because they are more likely to develop active disease.

Although no national data are available on the number of tuberculosis cases according to risk groups, some local estimates of the number of cases within these risk groups are available. In New York City, where rates of tuberculosis are about five times the national average, 20–30% of people with infectious tuberculosis are homeless; at least 40% are also infected with the human immunodeficiency virus (HIV); and a study conducted in The Bronx by the NYC Department of Health showed that more than 56% of tuberculosis patients reported drug and/or alcohol use.[10,12,19] According to the Centers for Disease Control (CDC), tuberculosis occurs at least three times more often in correctional settings than in the general population. In large correctional institutions, the incidence rate may be as high as 6 to 11 times that seen in the general population.[5]

The number of workers having prolonged contact with people known or suspected to have active tuberculosis, or with members of groups that are at high risk for tuberculosis is potentially enormous, especially in epidemic areas. Currently, more than 8.5 million health care workers and 1.9 million social service workers are employed in the United States.[1]

There has been a lag in the development of rapid methods for diagnosing TB infection and active tuberculosis disease. Methods for diagnosing tuberculosis infection remain stranded in the 19th century, with the purified protein derivative (PPD) tuberculin skin test as the only available method of identifying the presence of asymptomatic infection. Tuberculin testing is cumbersome and time-consuming, requires revisits, and, to be reliable, requires a functioning immune system. Those with immunosuppressive conditions, especially HIV infection, often show false negative reactions to the PPD tuberculin skin test but are more likely, once infected, to progress to active tuberculosis disease. These limitations can lead to increased worker exposure due to delayed diagnosis and may make screening of some workers ineffective.

Characteristics of the current epidemic—specifically, the intersection of the tuberculosis and HIV/AIDS epidemics and the emergence of tuberculosis strains that are resistant to multiple drugs (MDR-TB)—pose additional occupational risks. The methods for determining the susceptibility patterns of tuberculosis organisms require weeks to months to complete. Because patients infected with drug-resistant strains are likely to remain infectious longer, they pose a hazard to workers who provide services to them. As evidence of this, between 1989 and 1993 the CDC documented at least eight nosocomial outbreaks of MDR-TB in prisons and hospitals, which resulted in skin test conversions in more than 100 workers, at least 17 cases of MDR-TB and 6 deaths among workers, and about 300 reported nosocomial cases of transmission of MDR-TB to both patients and workers.[2,25]

Not until October 8, 1993, when OSHA promulgated national enforcement guidelines on tuberculosis control in the workplace,[24] has there been a legally enforceable basis for preventing occupational exposure to tuberculosis. These guidelines, while constituting an important advance, are new and relatively untested. Additionally, successful enforcement of these guidelines may be limited due to the scarcity of OSHA inspectors. For all these reasons, the current epidemic poses many challenges for preventing TB transmission in the workplace (as well as in the community). In the past, public and occupational health officials often successfully worked together to combat the disease. Yet, with the decline in tuberculosis rates, public health and occupational health efforts at TB control waned and diverged from each other.

HISTORICAL ROOTS

Early Epidemiology of Tuberculosis in the Workplace

During the late 19th and early 20th centuries, the combination of rapid industrial development, a burgeoning immigrant workforce, and the expansion of urban centers created a deplorable domestic and occupational context within which tuberculosis flourished.[27] Mortality data and workplace surveys in the United States showed that death from tuberculosis disproportionately affected low-wage workers.[15] At the 1906 Convention of the American Federation of Labor (AFL), TB was declared "labor's most pressing problem." The results of a survey of 53 occupations showed that marble and stone cutters, cigar makers, plasterers, printers, and servants were dying of tuberculosis at rates well above 4 per 1000 while bankers, brokers and "officials" had death rates below 1 per 1000.[28]

The identification of the tubercle bacillus in 1882 and the subsequent development and application of the tuberculin skin test meant that a method for widespread screening for tuberculosis infection was available. Eventually, the ability to diagnose tuberculosis infection led to workplace screening programs that documented high rates of infection among many occupational groups. The first reported screening of American workers for tuberculosis was conducted in 1908; among 203 printers studied, 34 (17%) were found to have active tuberculosis.[16] A 1913 study by the newly formed U.S. Public Health Service Division of Industrial Hygiene and Sanitation identified tuberculosis as "the most important and serious disease from which garment workers suffer." The study found that the TB prevalence rate among garment workers in New York City was 10 times that of US Army personnel. Disease rates were highest among garment workers in the lowest paying jobs, living in the smallest dwellings, with the largest number of household members.[30]

A 1915 study of tuberculosis conducted among 19,932 workers in Cincinnati in 38 different industries categorized the primary causes of the 220 active cases of tuberculosis (1.1%) as follows: "history of tuberculosis in the family (34%); working conditions (19%); poverty and poor housing (11%); venereal disease (7%); other diseases and injuries (6%); none of the above factors in special evidence (23%)."[26]

Taken together, the results of these early workplace screening programs identified *both* workplace and community risks for TB. Disease rates were consistently higher among workers in lower-paying jobs and having poor working and living conditions: poverty, overcrowding, bad housing, inadequate medical care. Given the types of industrial occupations surveyed, the results suggested that it was often not the intrinsic nature of job tasks per se (such as providing services to persons with TB) that posed an increased risk, but living and working in close contact with persons having active TB. People at highest risk faced multiple risk factors: at home (living in close quarters and poor housing), in the community (living in areas with high endemic rates of TB), and in the workplace (crowded and poorly ventilated).

Early Control Efforts

The identification of the causative organism and the prevalence of tuberculosis infection revealed by PPD testing gave added momentum to reform movements, which since the mid 1800s had been dedicated to improving the conditions of the working poor. The discovery that tuberculosis was communicable and the identification of the etiologic agent provided reformers with a definite enemy that could be vanquished, it was believed, by eliminating the poor housing, unsanitary factory conditions, and the unhygienic practices of the working poor.[9,27] During the same period, several union campaigns to make shop conditions more sanitary were linked to broad public health efforts in the battle against infectious disease.

Cleaning up the workplace and keeping the work force healthy were seen as beneficial to the worker, the employer, and the public.[28]

In the 1890s, under the leadership of Dr. Hermann Biggs, the New York City Department of Health developed the first comprehensive tuberculosis control program. Case finding, mandatory reporting, TB education for homes, schools, and factories, and a system of clinics, hospitals, nursing follow-up, and free laboratory testing were integrated within Biggs's system. One of the most controversial aspects of Biggs's tuberculosis control strategies, the mandatory removal of infectious tuberculosis patients to public hospitals, was influenced by Biggs's recognition of the potential for occupational transmission. Because disability and unemployment insurance were nonexistent, it was common for symptomatic workers with tuberculosis to cling to their jobs for as long as their strength held out. Biggs used the occupational hazard posed by this situation to justify the exercise of legal authority to move people with tuberculosis from work to treatment facilities.[29]

Shifting of Occupational and Public Health Efforts

Beginning in the mid 19th century, national tuberculosis mortality rates began declining in the United States,[27] with periodic peaks, particularly in urban areas, coinciding with the arrival of large numbers of immigrant poor.[8] It was not until the 1950s that CDC began collecting national data on the incidence of TB. These statistics also reveal a steady decline in the numbers of new cases: from 84,300 in 1953 to 22,000 in 1985. However, even during this period of overall decline, higher than average rates persisted in the poorest urban areas in Miami, Houston, Atlanta, and New York City. For example, in New York City in 1980, the overall age-adjusted incidence of TB was 19.9 per 100,000 population, but was roughly four times higher (78.6 per 100,000) in central Harlem.[20]

The overall decline in tuberculosis is generally attributed to the simultaneous improvement in public health interventions (case finding, contact tracing, establishment of diagnostic clinics, isolation of TB patients in sanatoria, pasteurization of milk) and better social conditions (improved nutrition and housing).[28] The decrease in tuberculosis mortality (case fatality rate) became marked with the widespread use of anti-tuberculosis medications.

With the decline in tuberculosis rates in the United States, public and occupational health control efforts shifted into new and divergent areas. In occupational health, despite an early focus on infectious disease, the subsequent emphasis has largely centered on chemical and physical hazards in the workplace. For example, a major initiative during the early part of the century was the establishment of workers' compensation systems to provide a means of support to workers who became disabled on the job. Nearly all of the awards made under workers' compensation were, and are still, the result of workplace injuries. This system has been inadequate for addressing the vast majority of workers afflicted with occupational diseases, infectious or otherwise.[14]

State and federal agencies responsible for occupational health and safety focused, by and large, on chemical hazards. As evidence of this, of the more than 59,000 substances on the National Institute for Occupational Safety and Health's (NIOSH) *Registry of Toxic Effects of Chemical Substances,* the Occupational Safety and Health Administration (OSHA), which is responsible for setting workplace standards, has set permissible exposure limits for fewer than 500 and detailed standards for fewer than 30 hazardous substances. Only one, the bloodborne pathogen standard, promulgated in 1992, specifically focuses on infectious agents.[6] The lack of attention to occupational health and safety in health care settings was documented by a 1970s NIOSH study that found that only 8% of more than 2,600 surveyed hospitals met all criteria for a comprehensive health and safety program.[17]

Likewise, after World War II, public health resources and attention began shifting away from TB control and into new areas. The widespread introduction of antibiotics in controlling infectious diseases, particularly in children and young adults, increased life expectancy. As large numbers of people began to survive to older ages, chronic, noncommunicable diseases such as cancer, cardiovascular, and renal disease increasingly captured the attention of public health officials. This shift is reflected in a 1950 policy statement of the American Public Health Association:

> Because of the marked changes in the age distribution of the population and in the spectrum of our health problems, the theory and practice of public health has been expanded. . . . The 'desirable minimal functions' of local health departments—vital statistics, sanitation, communicable disease control, laboratory services, maternal and child health and health education—have been modified recently to include the control of chronic diseases.[31]

THE CURRENT CRISIS

Public health, focused on chronic illness and lulled by the antibiotic era, and occupational health, focused on safety and chemical hazards, were unprepared for the emergence of HIV and AIDS in the early 1980s and for the reemergence of TB. After several decades of steady decline, the incidence of TB began to increase in 1985. From 1985 to 1990, the number of TB cases reported to the Centers for Disease Control rose by almost 16%, from 22,201 to 25,702 cases. The largest increases occurred in large urban areas and in 25- to 44-year-olds. As outbreaks of tuberculosis involving workers and patients in health care settings were reported,[3] the new epidemic, coming hard on the heels of the HIV epidemic, aroused public awareness about infectious disease and provoked concern about the dangers of contracting a serious infectious disease in the workplace.

Public Health and Occupational Health Approaches to Disease Control

We have already touched on some of the difficulties for disease control posed by the new epidemic: the myriad social and medical problems among the populations at greatest risk; the emergence of multidrug-resistant strains; and the lack of a quick, effective screening tool. Additional challenges emerge for controlling the transmission of TB in the workplace.

Although both public health and occupational health have a long history of disease control and prevention, each currently operates from different and sometimes competing legal, philosophical, and methodologic bases. It is useful to explore some of the similarities and differences and to examine the ways in which they are beginning to be addressed in recent initiatives.

LEGAL AND PHILOSOPHICAL BASIS

Public health laws mandate that local and state public health authorities take whatever steps are necessary to control disease and protect the public's health. The control of communicable diseases such as tuberculosis was one of the earliest functions of local health departments and remains today at the core of public health regulation. The key provisions are essentially those established by Biggs and include mandatory reporting, case and contact investigation, education, and procedures to prevent or control disease in people with the disease, their contacts, and carriers. Public health law is very clear that the societal need to protect the public's health, when a person endangers the health of others, may at times supersede individual liberties. (For example, see the New York City Health Code.[21])

By contrast, occupational health is generally regulated by federal and state departments of labor. The Occupational Safety and Health Act of 1970 imposes on private sector employers a *general duty* to provide a place of employment that is free from recognized hazards likely to cause death or serious physical harm to employees, and to comply with occupational safety and health standards promulgated and enforced under OSHA.[23] When employers fail to comply voluntarily, employees have the right to request government intervention. Implicit in this mandate is a recognition that the employer-employee relationship is not a democratic one. Occupational health laws attempt to ameliorate some of this inherent imbalance by providing workers with legal mechanisms to address health and safety hazards on the job.

Thus, while public health law reflects broad public health concerns such as the need to control TB, occupational health law serves a *mediating* role in labor/management conflicts over health and safety conditions.

There are also philosophical differences between public health and occupational health concerning the degree of hazard or risk that should be tolerated. The traditions of public health, nursing, and medicine are rooted in the fabled self-sacrifice and heroism of brave, pre-antibiotic era role models such as Florence Nightingale. As part of this tradition, the ethos of nursing, medical, and other health professional training is the transcendence of personal concerns in order to meet patients' needs. Students receive the message that some degree of infectious disease risk is unavoidable and must be tolerated as part of the job.

By contrast, the guiding principle in occupational health is to ensure that workplaces are safe. One clear reflection of this is embodied in NIOSH's mandate to "develop criteria . . . which will describe exposure levels . . . at which no worker will suffer impaired health or functional capacities or diminished life expectancy as a result of his [or her] work experience."[23] These are two very different principles: accepting that some degree of risk is inevitable vs. the idea that workplace conditions should pose no risk to employee health.

Philosophical differences regarding risk have become manifest in practical differences in the control of TB in the workplace. For example, some public health personnel assert that zero risk to workers is not a feasible goal in many health care or other settings serving large numbers of TB patients. Furthermore, it has been argued that were employers and employees to do all that is necessary to achieve zero risk in these settings, patient care and public health goals would be jeopardized.

In 1992, NIOSH recommended the use of powered high-efficiency particulate air (HEPA) filter half-mask respirators in situations where the potential for exposure to aerosolized droplet nuclei was considered to be "medium" (operating rooms, ICUs) or "indeterminant" (emergency rooms, waiting areas).[18] This recommendation was based on documented occurrences of occupational TB transmission and the recognition that prevailing guidelines[13] regarding particulate respirators were not adequate to prevent such transmssion. The use of "Darth Vader" type equipment was viewed with alarm by some public health personnel, who were concerned that the goal of engaging patients in long-term treatment appeared to be threatened by devices that might alienate patients already feeling stigmatized by the disease.[4]

In addition, many facilities that treat TB patients are public institutions, where funds are scarce. There is often reluctance to divert the limited money available from direct patient services to personal protective equipment. However, employees who feel unsafe at work cannot work effectively. For public health aims to be advanced, it is important that workers feel comfortable with and not fearful of their work environment.

Risk Assessment

Not only are there similarities and differences in the legal and philosophical bases of public health and occupational health, but similarities and differences exist in each discipline's approach to assessing what level of hazard is present and what mechanisms should be implemented to control it.

The concept of risk assessment is common to both occupational and public health practice. Both disciplines use risk indicators—such as the level of a particular contaminant in air or the infection rates in a population—to determine the level of risk. These indicators are then measured against a reference, guideline, or background rate to determine whether the levels are excessive. Results that fall within a standard or guideline are generally interpreted by governmental and managerial entities to mean that customary public and occupational health efforts to reduce or eliminate the hazard should continue but that no specific new intervention is necessary. Unusual measurements indicating excess risk demand attention in the form of increased efforts or new approaches to the hazard in question.

When applied to TB in the workplace, traditional approaches to risk assessment are problematic. In occupational health, the standard approach to measuring hazards is through monitoring environmental exposures. The measured level of contaminants is compared with standards or guidelines set forth by recognized regulatory or advisory entities. Because the concentration of TB organisms in the environment cannot be measured, there are no practical analogues to environmental exposure monitoring in tuberculosis control. The best available approaches to evaluating the degree of workplace risk are indirect: the evaluation of infection control practices, environmental controls, and PPD conversion rates among employees. At this time, the monitoring of PPD conversion rates of employees within and among (comparable) institutions, over time, is the most relied-upon method for evaluating tuberculosis control practices. This method is far from ideal for protection of worker health, since infection must occur before unsafe working conditions are identified.

One important issue arising from this approach is the criteria for determining whether there is an "excess" level of risk or number of conversions in a workplace where there are people with known or suspected TB. Should even one conversion in a workplace where TB patients are treated be cause for concern? Or, must there be a "cluster" of two or more conversions within a certain time frame? Or, must conversion rates exceed previous rates or exceed rates where there is no occupational exposure? Does this depend on how many TB patients are treated in the facility—or on the background rate of infection and disease in the surrounding community? Can a numerical standard be set that will be applicable to all settings? Clearly, the choice of evaluation criteria will influence the results of the risk assessment:

whether a risk of occupational TB transmission is deemed to exist, what the magnitude of that risk is, and what interventions are necessary.

Also, evaluating conversion rates requires collecting data over relatively long times, generally for months or years. Because the PPD skin test is dependent on a functioning immune system, the current prevalence of HIV infection creates the possibility of false negatives within populations for whom accurate results are critical. At best, PPD testing can only provide an assessment of prior but not necessarily of present risk.

Finally, there is a question about which workers are really at risk. Both occupational and public health officials emphasize that occupational transmission of tuberculosis has been documented and is a potential threat to workers in health care settings, prisons, shelters for the homeless, drug treatment centers, and long-term care facilities. These workers, depending on local epidemiologic conditions, have repeated, prolonged contact with high-risk groups, direct contact with infectious TB patients, and may perform high-hazard procedures such as bronchoscopy, aerosolized pentamidine treatment, sputum induction, suction procedures, or autopsies.[22,24]

Additional concerns about occupational transmission of TB have been raised in settings such as soup kitchens, income maintenance centers, and social service agencies, where the population served and not the service provided constitutes a potential transmission risk. Little is known about the actual risk of occupational tuberculosis transmission in these settings. Without information about PPD conversion rates in nonclinical, possibly-at-risk settings, it is difficult to effectively allocate resources. Those responsible for public health and occupational health need to know more about the risk of occupationally acquired tuberculosis infection and disease among employees serving people who are epidemiologically at risk for tuberculosis.

Risk Management and Control

Both occupational health and public health employ a hierarchy of methods and procedures to control disease. In the hierarchy, methods of control that involve the highest potential for prevention and are least subject to human error are preferable to measures that are undertaken to contain and treat the disease after exposure and transmission have occurred.

In occupational health, the hierarchy of controls is aimed at preventing *exposure.* Proceeding from most to least preferable, these control methods are as follows:

1. Substituting less hazardous materials for hazardous ones
2. Preventing the release or build-up of hazardous materials in the worker's environment by isolating the source and using engineering controls such as ventilation or shielding
3. Limiting contact between worker and hazard by administrative methods such as exclusion of all but essential personnel from isolation rooms, rapid triage of emergency room patients who are coughing, the requirement that anyone observed coughing in a clinic waiting room wear a mask
4. The use of personal protective equipment such as respirators, gowns, gloves. Personal protective devices, because they have little effect on ultimate source control aims and because they place the burden of control upon the worker, rank lowest on the hierarchy of controls.

The hierarchy of controls guiding public health policy is as follows:

1. Primary prevention is aimed at inhibiting the development of disease. In TB control, this means preventing the transmission of the organism from an

infectious individual to others through the rapid identification, isolation, and complete treatment of persons with active TB. Case finding, mandatory reporting of cases, contact investigation procedures, and appropriate TB prophylaxis are essential to primary prevention efforts.

2. Secondary prevention involves reducing the consequences of disease through early detection and treatment. Secondary prevention in tuberculosis control includes not only therapy for tuberculosis disease but also identification, through PPD screening, of those who are *infected* so that preventive therapy can be used to reduce the likelihood that tuberculosis infection will progress to disease.

3. Tertiary prevention, promoting the optimum functioning of people already affected by disease, including promoting the completion of treatment, is accomplished by improved access to medical supervision, housing, and social services.[17] In the case of tuberculosis control, tertiary prevention through completion of treatment also serves a primary prevention function.

SOLUTIONS: FORGING THE LINK

Both occupational and public health approaches are necessary for controlling TB in the workplace. Primary prevention must be the overriding goal of tuberculosis control efforts in the workplace and in the community. Tuberculosis can effectively be reduced by early detection, isolation, and complete treatment of tuberculosis patients and by treating such patients within environments where adequate engineering, administrative, and personal protective measures are in place. In the absence of direct monitoring methods for tuberculosis organisms, PPD surveillance is the best quantitative method available to assess risk.

Such a comprehensive approach is embodied in the CDC's draft *Guidelines for Preventing the Transmission of Tuberculosis in Health Care Facilities.*[5] The guidelines establish minimum requirements for TB control programs in *all* health care facilities. They include initial and periodic risk assessment; a written infection control program; assignment of responsibility for the program to qualified individuals; procedures for prompt identification, isolation and management of people known or suspected to have TB; implementing and monitoring engineering controls; respiratory protection; education, counseling, and screening of health care workers; and evaluation of skin test data.

The protocol for risk assessment includes a method of quantifying risk within specific settings using both PPD conversion rates and the number of infectious patients treated within specific areas of the facility. Based on the results of ongoing risk assessment, additional controls may be required. The new CDC approach is extremely localized: It enables institutions to define risk and to prescribe responses in accordance with the clinical and PPD experience of discrete areas within institutions. This approach recognizes that the likelihood of exposure to tuberculosis depends on local prevalence of tuberculosis.

At the same time, these guidelines—while combining key control strategies from both occupational and public health—will not immediately ensure that occupational exposure to TB is prevented. Below we review some of the outstanding issues and additional recommendations for addressing them.

First, in addition to involving people with expertise in infection control, occupational health, and engineering in the development and implementation of TB control programs, such individuals also need to be involved in the resource allocation process. Despite, or perhaps because of, the recent increases in federal funding for tuberculosis control, it is extremely difficult to achieve a consensus of opinion about resource allocation. There are numerous competing demands for TB resources: screening and medical follow-up, surveillance, DOT, ventilation. Ideally, money should be spent on all these things, but how much and in what proportions?

Given that public health funding is limited, what money is available must be applied to maximum effect. Epidemiologic surveillance, through monitoring of PPD skin test conversion rates and the rates of active disease, will ultimately enable public and occupational health personnel to prudently deploy resources and to monitor the efficacy of existing control measures. In the meantime, as a priority, engineering, administrative and personal protective controls *must* be implemented in settings and during procedures in which the risk of tuberculosis transmission is clearly a possibility. One way to begin making these decisions on a more rational basis is to bring all of the players and expertise to the decision-making process.

Second, some recommendations, although logical and in line with good occupational health and public health practice, have not been adequately demonstrated to be effective. Systematic evaluation and ongoing monitoring in field settings is required in order to assess the efficacy of specific engineering controls, such as modular HEPA units, germicidal ultraviolet irradiation, and the optimum number of air changes. It is not yet known which combination of controls is most effective in reducing TB transmission. Therefore, funding and research on the use of these controls, linked to PPD surveillance data, is sorely needed.

Third, specific recommendations concerning respiratory protection appropriate to specific circumstances, in conjunction with a plan to collect reliable data, are needed. Personal protective devices are absolutely essential in many clinical settings where tuberculosis patients are treated. But confusion and disagreement remains about the type and level of respiratory protection that is necessary under different circumstances.

Fourth, the CDC guidelines are designed for health care and other clinical facilities. As mentioned above, risk assessment for and control of TB in nonclinical settings where services are provided to epidemiologically high-risk individuals remains problematic. The number and variety of such settings is potentially great. From the public health perspective, allocating resources for PPD screening in low incidence areas of the country, or in nonclinical settings where there is no demographic reason to assume that the risk of tuberculosis transmission exists, seems wasteful. In such settings standard public health methods, specifically contact investigation, should serve to identify people infected with and exposed to tuberculosis so that targeted PPD testing can be conducted. While this approach has the advantage of being both focused upon and adaptable to local conditions, it does not answer the question about the real risk in these settings, nor does it provide any information or current protection for people who work in them.

One way of addressing this would be through a combination of tuberculosis education for workers and mandated screening in specific settings where geography, demographics, or epidemiology indicates that risk exists. In addition, pilot PPD surveillance programs of representative settings where the risk is assumed but unknown should be conducted. This approach should be coupled with careful environmental evaluation and, ideally, should also include baseline screening of the served population for tuberculosis symptoms and history. The screening process, whch can be conducted by lay people, can identify people who may have active tuberculosis and will serve the purpose of taking possibly infectious people from the general population to a clinical setting for evaluation. This approach could provide information about the numbers of tuberculosis patients served and provide managers of nonclinical settings with risk assessment data analogous to that recommended in the current draft CDC guidelines for clinical settings. Such an approach could lead to informed policy decisions about risk assessment and risk management methods in nonclinical settings.

CONCLUSION

In the early part of the 20th century, social reform efforts were aimed at improving the conditions of working people at home and in the workplace. Many trade unions successfully gained workers' compensation, medical care, and insurance benefits as protection against economic insecurity.[27] The tuberculosis epidemic of the 1990s, following hard on the heels of the HIV/AIDS epidemic, will require research and collaboration to reach agreement among public health, labor, and occupational health. Despite differences between these groups, the solution, voiced by a Public Health Service official more than 75 years ago, still applies today: "[Hygienic] conditions in [the workplace] must be considered as forming a part of the general field of public health . . . [workplace] conditions affecting the health of the worker can never be separated from those of his total environment, nor is it possible to define where the field of industrial hygiene ceases and public health begins."[30]

REFERENCES

1. Bureau of Labor Statistics: Current Employment Statistics, 1992 Annual Averages. Washington, DC, US Dept of Labor.
2. Centers for Disease Control: Guidelines for preventing the transmission of tuberculosis in health care settings, with special focus on HIV-related issues. 39(RR-17):1–29, 1990.
3. Centers for Disease Control: Nosocomial transmission of multidrug-resistant tuberculosis to health care workers and HIV-infected patients in an urban hospital—Florida. MMWR 39:718–722, 1990.
4. Centers for Disease Control: Issues in preventing tuberculosis transmission in health care facilities [meeting]. Atlanta, October 22–23, 1992.
5. Centers for Disease Control: Control of tuberculosis in correctional facilities: A guide for health care workers. Atlanta, 1992.
6. Centers for Disease Control: 29 CFR 1910.1030, July 1993.
7. Centers for Disease Control: Draft guidelines for preventing the transmission of tuberculosis in health care facilities, 2nd ed; Notice of comment period. Federal Register 58:52810–52853, October 12, 1993.
8. Drolet GJ, Lowell AM: A Half Century's Progress Against Tuberculosis in New York City, 1900–1950. New York, Tuberculosis and Health Association, 1952.
9. Dubos R, Dubos J: The White Plague: Tuberculosis, Man, and Society. New Brunswick, NJ, Rutgers State University, 1987.
10. Eaton C, Rubino M: New York City Department of Health, 1993 (unpublished data).
11. Hamburg M: Strengthening the infrastructure for public health in the United States. Presented at the World Congress on Tuberculosis, Bethesda, MD, November 16–19, 1992.
12. Hinman A: Personal communication. Centers for Disease Control and Prevention, August 4, 1993.
13. Markowitz SB, Fischer E, Fahs MC, et al: Occupational disease in New York state: A comprehensive examination. Am J Ind Med 16:417–435, 1989.
14. Mausner J, Kramer S: Mausner & Bahn Epidemiology: An Introductory Text. 2nd ed. Philadelphia, WB Saunders, 1985.
15. Miller JA: Pulmonary tuberculosis among printers. Proceedings of the Sixth International Congress on Tuberculosis, Vol 3, p 209.
16. Morgan JW: Concise Epidemiology: A Practical Text. Bryn Mawr, CA, MDM Consulting, 1991.
17. National Institute for Occupational Safety and Health: Hospital occupational services study, 1974–1976, Vol 1–7: 1975–1976. Cincinnati, NIOSH, US Dept of Health and Human Services publication NIOSH 75-101.

18. National Institute for Occupational Safety and Health: Recommended guidelines for personal respiratory protection of workers in health care facilities potentially exposed to tuberculosis. Atlanta, September 14, 1992.
19. New York City Department of Health: Tuberculosis in New York, City Information Summary, 1991.
20. New York City Department of Health: Tuberculosis in New York, City Information Summary, 1992.
21. New York City Health Code, Article 11: Reportable Diseases and Conditions. Rules of the City of New York, June 30, 1991.
22. New York State Department of Labor Public Employee Safety and Health Program: Enforcement guidelines for occupational exposure to tuberculosis, April 17, 1992.
23. Occupational Safety and Health Act of 1970, 29 USC. Washington, DC.
24. Occupational Safety and Health Administration: Enforcement policy and procedures for occupational exposure to tuberculosis, October 8, 1993.
25. Occupational Safety and Health Administration, Region II: Enforcement guidelines for occupational exposure to tuberculosis, October 10, 1993.
26. Robinson DE, Wilson JG: Tuberculosis among industrial workers. Public Health Bulletin #73, Washington, DC, Government Printing Office, 1916.
27. Rosen G: Preventive Medicine in the United States, 1900–1975. New York, Prodist, 1977.
28. Rosner D, Markowitz G (eds): Dying for Work: Workers' Safety and Health in Twentieth Century America. Bloomington, IN, Indiana University Press, 1987.
29. Rothman S: The sanitorium experience. In The TB Revival: Individual Rights and Societal Obligations in a Time of AIDS. New York, United Hospital Fund, 1993.
30. Schereschewsky: The health of garment workers. In Studies in Vocational Diseases, Public Health Bulletin #71. Washington, DC, Government Printing Office, 1915.
31. The local health department—Services and responsibilities. Am J Public Health 41:302–307, 1951.
32. Voelker R: TB control guidelines cause coast-to-coast confusion. American Medical News 36(6):1, 56, 1993.

JAMES MELIUS, MD, DrPH
DEBORAH NAGIN, MPH

FUTURE NEEDS: RESEARCH, EDUCATION, AND SERVICE

From the Division of Occupational Health and Environmental Epidemiology
New York State Department of Health
Albany, New York

Reprint requests to:
James Melius, MD, DrPH
Director
Division of Occupational Health and Environmental Epidemiology
New York State Department of Health
2 University Place
Room 350
Albany, NY 12203-3399

The reemergence of tuberculosis as a major public health problem in the United States has also led to its resurgence as a significant occupational health problem for people in many different occupations.[3] As illustrated elsewhere in this volume, the epidemic of TB potentially affects people working in many different settings, and controlling the risk of tuberculosis for workers in some of these settings may be very difficult. Control of the workplace risk largely depends on control of the disease in the community. However, our current capabilities in occupational disease prevention should allow better control of tuberculosis transmission in health care facilities and other settings while the community epidemic is being controlled.

This chapter will discuss some of the efforts needed to control the workplace transmission of tuberculosis. While the chapter is divided into sections on research, education, and service, divisions between these categories are not distinct. Better preventive services need not await "definitive" results from research before being implemented. We must do what we can now while we await better information. To emphasize that approach, the chapter has been organized to first discuss what research is needed and then to discuss what can be done in the meantime.

RESEARCH NEEDS

The current tuberculosis epidemic has made the health care community acutely aware of the many gaps in knowledge about tuberculosis control measures.[8] The relatively low rate of tuberculosis infection in the United States in the recent past meant that most health care facilities did not need to place a high priority on the prevention of transmission of tuberculosis. Much more attention was paid to the prevention of bloodborne infections and to other types of infection control problems. However, the reemergence of tuberculosis has forced health care facilities to reassess priorities and allocate more money and manpower to help reduce the risk of transmission.

The following items represent major research needs for the control of tuberculosis in the workplace.

Identification of Infectious Patients

The prompt and accurate identification of infectious patients is critical for the prevention of the transmission of airborne infections in health care facilities. More sensitive and faster techniques for detecting tubercle bacilli on smears and cultures are currently being developed and introduced.[1,9] This capability should provide better identification and quicker implementation of isolation procedures. More rapid identification of drug-resistant organisms is also important. The ability to identify the degree of infectiousness of a particular patient would also be very helpful. Current methods of evaluation only provide a relatively crude indicator of infectiousness, and current control procedures essentially assume that all identified patients are equally infectious. However, some patients are much more infectious than others, and methods to determine the degree of infectiousness would indicate the need for additional or stricter control measures for such patients.

After treatment has started, it is also important to know when a patient is no longer infectious. Although this determination may be similar to identifying an infectious patient, different considerations of sensitivity and specificity may apply, and a rapid test may not be as critical (but would still be helpful). This information will be particularly important for decisions relating to the discharge of infected patients from hospitals.

Techniques for Measuring Airborne Concentration of TB

A method to determine airborne levels of TB would be very helpful in order to evaluate current and new control measures. This would allow the evaluation of different ventilation designs and the effectiveness of other control approaches such as high-efficiency particulate air (HEPA) filters. The potential risk in different areas in health care facilities could also be evaluated better. Without such a quantification technique, PPD conversion rates must be used to monitor the effectiveness of control techniques, and it is difficult to determine which part of the control program was effective. It should be feasible to develop a method for measuring airborne concentrations of TB with polymerase chain reaction or other techniques and then to apply that technique in the evaluation of control measures.

Assessment of the Effectiveness of Ultraviolet Light Disinfection

Ultraviolet light irradiation appears to be a very effective control technique and may be the only feasible engineering control measure for many settings (e.g., waiting rooms).[7] However, there is some skepticism about its effectiveness, and little information is available to determine (1) the design and operational parameters to ensure proper air circulation across the lamp and (2) the impact of high humidity and other factors that may limit the effectiveness of UV.

Follow-up Studies in Hospitals

Much of the recently available data on the transmission of tuberculosis in hospitals have been derived from epidemics among health care facility employees and patients.[2,4] In nearly all of these situations, many different aspects of the control programs have broken down, making it difficult to isolate the relative efficacy of individual control procedures. Currently, large numbers of workers in health care and related facilities are being exposed to tuberculosis and other airborne infections. Follow-up studies of these workers are needed to better understand the sources of airborne infections and the efficacy of current control procedures.

Other Settings

Employees who work in health care facilities other than hospitals, such as outpatient clinics, or who work in facilities that provide services to people at high risk of developing tuberculosis, such as homeless shelters and drug treatment centers, may also be at risk from the transmission of tuberculosis. There is very little information on the risk of transmission in these settings or on the applicability and effectiveness of TB control measures. Even though the risk of tuberculosis transmission may be less than the risk associated with isolation rooms or high-risk procedure areas, control of transmission may be much more difficult due to the problems in recognizing and "isolating" infectious clients. This situation is particularly problematic in settings without readily available health care expertise. Control approaches such as ultraviolet lights and HEPA filters are promising, but evaluation of the effectiveness and applicability of these and other control measures is needed.

Respirators

The type of respirator to be used to prevent transmission of tuberculosis has been one of the most contentious issues in relation to tuberculosis control guidelines. Regardless of the financial considerations, this debate has pointed out the need for better research on respirator performance for protection from bioaerosols and for the development of more comfortable respirators that do not interfere with communication and vision.

Ventilation

The primary method for preventing transmission from infectious patients has been the use of isolation rooms. Even though isolation rooms have been used for many years, there has been very little research on the efficacy of different parameters of the design and operation of these units. Issues such as design of anterooms, ventilation rates, and ventilation flow patterns need to be evaluated.

Vaccination

The development of good immunization methods could be the most effective method for preventing transmission to workers in health care facilities. Health care workers in some countries are routinely given bacille Calmette-Guérin vaccine to protect against tuberculosis. However, the efficacy of BCG for the protection of employees from TB transmission is unclear.[5,6] This issue needs to be reevaluated and better methods developed.

EDUCATION

Perhaps the most important part of TB control programs will be the training and education of the thousands of workers potentially affected by transmission of tuberculosis within their workplace settings. Many control measures to prevent tuberculosis transmission are dependent on proper work practices such as isolation procedures. Training of the involved workers will be critical to the proper implementation of these practices.

People who potentially need training can be divided into four categories: workers in hospitals, in other health care facilities, other settings, and workers in related occupations.

Hospitals

Workers in hospitals are at greatest risk for TB transmission. Due to the higher risk of exposure and the complexities of controlling transmission in such facilities, these employees will need a significant amount of training about risks and the specific approaches the hospital is using to control them. Many different groups of employees within a hospital will need training about their specific risks, and they will also need some knowledge of the preventive steps and procedures being used for other groups of workers. This training needs to be continually updated to reflect changes in the types of patients potentially infected with TB and changes in control procedures.

Other Health Care Facilities

People working in other types of health care facilities, such as outpatient clinics or patients' homes, will be at some risk for transmission of TB. However, greater emphasis will need to be placed on the recognition and appropriate referral of potentially infectious patients rather than on specific isolation room procedures.

Other Workplace Settings

Due to the nature of the current TB epidemic, some people working in settings unrelated to health care will occasionally be at risk for TB due to the infection of a fellow worker or other contact with an infectious person. In some situations the risk may be very low, but other places of employment may provide services to people at high risk of TB infection or may employ people from geographic regions with a high incidence of TB. People in all of these settings will need prompt follow-up that includes counseling about their potential health risk, follow-up procedures, and other aspects of infection control.

Related Occupations

Many types of professional groups will need training about tuberculosis control, including industrial hygienists, occupational medicine physicians, occupational health nurses, architects, and ventilation engineers. Educational programs specific to the individual groups and interdisciplinary training sessions should both be presented.

SERVICE

In one sense, the description of the needs for services for the prevention of tuberculosis transmission is simple. Current guidelines from the Centers for Disease Control, the Occupational Safety and Health Administration, and other groups address the prevention of transmission. While quarrels abound about certain aspects of these guidelines, they do provide a sound basis for preventive programs. We simply need to implement these guidelines. Areas that should be emphasized are described below.

Identifying Infectious Patients

The experience in New York and other areas makes it clear that much needs to be done to improve the identification of TB-infected patients in health care facilities. This includes better availability of diagnostic services and better protocols for identifying potentially infectious patients in different parts of the health care system. For settings such as emergency departments, this can be accomplished through protocols for the identification of potentially infected patients and the subsequent implementation of special procedures for isolating and providing more rapid diagnostic testing for these patients. This type of approach needs to be extended to other types of facilities that care for "high-risk" patients, such as extended care facilities, home health care, and homeless shelters.

Isolation Rooms and Other Physical Plant Changes

Hospitals in New York City and other areas with a large increase in the incidence of tuberculosis have not had adequate isolation facilities to handle the number of patients requiring isolation. An adequate number of isolation rooms need to be built to address the potential need.

High-Risk Procedures

Protecting health care personnel during special procedures such as sputum induction and bronchoscopy is critical due to the high risk of transmission from these procedures. Enhanced ventilation, development of safer work procedures, and appropriate respiratory protection need to be implemented to reduce TB transmission in these procedure areas.

Surveillance Programs

Health care and other facilities with an increased risk of tuberculosis transmission need to have good tuberculosis surveillance programs for their employees. These programs are important for facilities with both a high risk and lower risk of transmission. Only through good surveillance will risk be identifiable in low-risk settings. Surveillance programs must follow sound practices and should include standard follow-up procedures for all employees whose skin tests convert to positive. All of these programs must include analysis of the medical surveillance results to identify conversion patterns by location, job title, and other factors.

Surveillance systems also must be instituted through local and state health departments so that they can identify infected patients and share this information with health care providers. Surveillance systems also will allow the identification of workplace settings with an increased incidence of tuberculosis infection among employees for evaluation and follow-up.

Workers' Compensation

We must address the problems of employees who will be infected with tuberculosis because of the failure of preventive programs. These employees may be at risk not only for acute illness but also for the development of active disease many years later. Appropriate follow-up programs must be provided for these workers as well as appropriate compensation without endless challenges to these claims. For example, the establishment of presumptive risk for health care workers in certain high-risk settings would eliminate unnecessary disputes about responsibility for medical bills and help to ensure adequate long-term follow-up of infected employees.

CONCLUSION

The prevention of the transmission of tuberculosis to workers in health care and other settings represents a major challenge in the field of occupational health. We must provide the money, personnel, and commitment to address this challenge.

REFERENCES

1. Abe C, Hosojima S, Fukasawa Y, et al: Comparison of MB-Check, BACTEC, and egg-based media for recovery of mycobacteria. J Clin Microbiol 30:878–881, 1992.
2. Beck-Sague C, Dooley SW, et al: Hospital outbreak of multidrug-resistant Mycobacterium tuberculosis infections. Factors in transmission to staff and HIV-infected persons. JAMA 268:1280–1286, 1992.
3. Centers for Disease Control: Guidelines for preventing the transmission of tuberculosis in health-care settings, with special focus on HIV-related issues. MMWR 39(RR–17):1–29, 1990.
4. Centers for Disease Control: Mycobacterium tuberculosis transmission in a health clinic—Florida, 1988. MMWR 38:256–264, 1989.
5. Collins FM: Tuberculosis: The return of an old enemy. Crit Rev Microbiol 19:1–16, 1993.
6. Lugosi L: Theoretical and methodological aspects of BCG vaccine from the discovery of Calmette and Guérin to molecular biology. A review. Tubercle Lung Dis 73:252–261, 1992.
7. Macher J: The use of germicidal lamps to control tuberculosis in healthcare facilities. Infect Control Hosp Epidemiol 14:723–728, 1993.
8. National Institute for Occupational Safety and Health: Proceedings of the Workshop on Engineering Controls for Preventing Airborne Infections in Workers in Health Care and Related Facilities. Cincinnati, NIOSH, 1994 (in press).
9. Wilson SM, McNerney R, Nye PM, et al: Progress toward a simplified polymerase chain reaction and its application to diagnosis of tuberculosis. J Clin Microbiol 31:776–782, 1993.

EDWARD ANSELM, MD

TUBERCULOSIS IN OFFICE SETTINGS: THE ANXIETY AND THE REALITY

From Empire Blue Cross and Blue Shield
New York, New York

Reprint requests to:
Edward Anselm, MD
Director, Employee Health Services
Empire Blue Cross and Blue Shield
622 Third Ave., Third Floor
New York, NY 10017

The office environment presents unique challenges to the early identification, evaluation, and resolution of tuberculosis outbreaks. With the increasing prevalence of tuberculosis, outbreaks in office settings are increasingly likely to occur. Compounding these issues are the heightened concerns regarding drug-resistant tuberculosis, anxieties about working with people who may have AIDS, and the generally unrealistic expectations many people have regarding the ability of medicine to provide definitive answers.

Workplace exposure to tuberculosis usually occurs in settings in which people with a likelihood of having active tuberculosis are likely to congregate. Hospitals, clinics, prisons, social service agencies, and shelters for the homeless are known to present significant risk to workers and visitors. In response to these well-understood risks, mandates have been developed that require these settings to provide varying degrees of environmental controls, protective equipment, and surveillance of workers.[2] As a result, workers and managers in these settings are prepared to deal with issues surrounding possible exposures. This stands in marked contrast to low-risk settings.

The low probability of tuberculosis occurring in office settings leads to neglect in developing policies and procedures to identify and evaluate potential outbreaks. The consequences of this type of neglect can be seen in the outbreak of drug-resistant tuberculosis at La Quinta High School in Westminster, California. Although not an office environment, this situation can be viewed as a worst case scenario. Twelve students developed active tuberculosis with a resistant strain, and 30% of the student body of 1,269 developed a positive skin test.[5]

A systematic approach to evaluation and resolution of potential and actual workplace tuberculosis outbreaks includes (1) early identification of potential or actual exposures, (2) screening for tuberculosis, and (3) appropriate communication with all employees. The following cases allow us to explore these issues further.

Case 1: The Mailroom

A 42-year-old mailroom employee developed hemoptysis and was taken from the mailroom by ambulance during the evening shift. The company's medical department was not notified. Seven weeks later a request for disability benefits was received by the medical department. At that point, the employee had been hospitalized and treated for active tuberculosis and was expected to be able to return to work within one week. Phone calls to the patient, treating physicians, the hospital infection control nurse, and the local tuberculosis control bureau verified the following facts: The patient had been sick for several weeks with cough, fever, chills, night sweats, and weight loss but had not sought medical attention. The patient was diagnosed as having a reactivation of old tuberculosis and responded quickly to standard therapy. Sputa from late in the hospital stay revealed no organisms, and the employees' symptoms resolved. Family members had been evaluated for tuberculosis, but neither the board of health nor the hospital infection control group had thought to call the employer.

Case 2: Claims Examiners

A human resources administrator of a remote office site called to inform the medical director that three individuals in the same claims review unit were found to have positive TB skin-test reactions. The site included 600 workers in three adjacent buildings. The physician's assistant treating all three was contacted. None of the individuals had active tuberculosis or recent disease. A review of records in the employee health service and at the county health department was conducted. No cases of active tuberculosis in employees, former employees, or temporary employees working at that location were identified.

The next day a newsletter explaining these recent events was distributed to all employees at that site along with an article on tuberculosis from the company magazine. The following day a fourth positive skin test was identified in the unit. Managers described the anxiety level as high. A decision was made to screen all employees in the affected unit and those who had routine business there. A clearly worded E-mail message was sent to all supervisors regarding the screening.

The next Monday, 150 of the 600 employees sought screening. Most of them had no routine business in the affected unit. PPD skin testing of the 40 employees who worked in or visited the unit was performed. The medical director read all of the skin tests 48 hours later. Each employee was privately interviewed and counseled. Positive skin reactions were found in two of the 40 employees, and neither of them had ever experienced symptoms of active tuberculosis during their employment with the company.

In the afternoon after the screening was completed, managers and supervisors met with the medical director to review the situation. Several of the supervisors came to the meeting convinced that the company must "do something" and would not listen to a reasonable presentation of the facts about tuberculosis and the meaning of information accumulated in the investigation. The position of the medical director and the county health department was that no further investigation was warranted by the facts. The discussion then shifted to how to deal with employee perceptions.

Case 3: Customer Service

A 50-year-old customer service representative was hospitalized with the diagnosis "rule out tuberculosis." She had experienced a chronic productive cough for several weeks and was found to have a positive PPD reaction. In the hospital, a bronchoscopy was performed, and the smear was AFB-negative. Because of the positive skin test the patient was placed on prophylactic therapy. The employee remained in continuous communication with the supervisor and coworkers, informing them that she was being treated for tuberculosis. However, no clarification regarding the lack of infectiousness to family and coworkers was provided.

EARLY IDENTIFICATION OF POTENTIAL EXPOSURES

When the index of suspicion for tuberculosis is low, the policies and procedures for providing management with early indications of possible exposure are frequently absent. Doctors' notes clearing individuals to return to work after medical illness frequently omit the diagnosis for reasons of confidentiality. With regard to tuberculosis, physicians assume that the local health department will trace contacts in the workplace. This is not always the case. Only 29 states specifically require contact investigation for reported cases of tuberculosis.[3] Therefore, some procedure for review of medical clearances may be in order. This procedure is usually in place in companies with an in-house medical department. Companies without a medical department may contract with occupational medicine clinics to obtain this service.

If an employee exhibits some of the symptoms of tuberculosis, referral for a medical evaluation may be warranted. Supervisors should be made aware of this possibility and have access to more expert personnel to discuss their concerns. If there is reasonable suspicion that active tuberculosis is present, a medical examination can be required. Workplaces have the right, if not the duty, to exclude such persons from the workplace until sufficient reassurances are obtained.[3] Policies and procedures for determining fitness for duty must include provisions for evaluation of infectious diseases. In developing and implementing these policies, significant attention must be paid to employee concerns about privacy and confidentiality, as well as labor relations issues.

If there is a concern regarding exposure in the workplace, appropriately trained personnel should be available to assemble the available information and assess the degree of risk. In the initial stages, concern may be driven by secondhand information. In the customer service scenario (case 3), neither the patient nor her treating physicians could be reached, and the hospital infection control nurse would not discuss the case for "reasons of confidentiality." In general, treating physicians will discuss the potential for the spread of active tuberculosis with other doctors, and in this instance a covering physician was able to explain that all sputa so far had been negative.

Part of the initial investigation involves identifying coworkers who may have had a significant exposure. In the mailroom (case 1), 24 workers sharing a relatively large mail sorting area were exposed to a person with active tuberculosis. As they worked an evening shift, there was no traffic through their work area. Thus, screening could be limited to the workers who had been potentially exposed. In some instances, such as the claims processing case (case 2), identifying potentially exposed persons (even though there was no exposure) was more complicated. A large number of employees, some in other buildings, felt that they had been exposed. Ultimately, a voluntary screening program was offered to help bring the matter to a close.

During an investigation, attention should be paid to the ventilation system. Areas receiving air from a source where active tuberculosis is present may be at risk. The investigator should use a low threshold for including employees with only occasional contact but can draw the line at the point of incidental contact in hallways or cafeterias. From the labor relations point of view, it would be prudent to be as inclusive as practical.

SCREENING FOR TUBERCULOSIS

Ideally, the decision to conduct screening of potentially exposed workers should be based on the clinical information available. The procedures for evaluation and follow-up of persons exposed to active tuberculosis are well known.[1] The optimal investigation of a workplace exposure should include a baseline PPD and symptom survey and a repeat PPD and symptom survey 10 weeks after the exposure. Rarely is an investigation so straightforward. In the mailroom case, the employer was not notified until 6 weeks after the last exposure. Thus, baseline PPD skin testing could not be performed, and the ability to accurately investigate the exposure was further limited by the finding of a large number of positive PPDs on first testing. Many of the mailroom employees were born in countries with a high prevalence of tuberculosis. Public health policy in their native countries requires childhood vaccination with bacille Calmette-Guérin vaccine, which results in positive PPD skin testing in about 50% of adults.[6] Employees already aware of a positive reaction were not tested.

The presence of positive PPD skin reactions at the onset of an investigation can confound efforts to educate employees about the significance of the exposure. Many physicians will resort to chest x-rays for evaluation of these patients. Although recommended for health care workers, the clinical significance of chest x-rays for people without symptoms is not clear.[1,4] If one routinely recommends prophylaxis with isoniazid for all people who have positive skin tests for tuberculosis, the question of recent versus past exposure in these patients is moot.

People with impaired T-cell immunity, such as those who are HIV-positive, present a special concern. Their response to the PPD antigen, even in the presence of active disease, is reduced or eliminated. Special sensitivity must be given to the privacy of HIV-positive people screened during workplace investigations. Because many such people are often unwilling to discuss their HIV status with the investigating health care workers, written materials provided to them and their physicians must be sufficiently broad to advise them of the special risk of tuberculosis for people who are HIV-positive. An even more difficult question involves people who are unaware of their HIV status. The most comprehensive approach would be to include counseling regarding the risks known to be associated with becoming HIV-positive and referral for outside testing for people who perceive themselves to be at risk.

Screening for tuberculosis should be offered free during working hours. A synopsis of the circumstances surrounding the exposure should be given to exposed workers so that, if they choose, they may pursue the advice of their personal physician. Although the additional investigation conducted by the private physician may have superfluous components (such as chest x-rays), the expense of this evaluation and any treatment recommended should be covered by Workers' Compensation. The employer cannot require participation in worksite tuberculosis exposure investigations unless the work setting is known to have an elevated risk for tuberculosis or the individual employee is thought to have active tuberculosis.[2,3]

Workers found to have converted from a negative to a positive PPD skin test should be advised to begin prophylaxis with isoniazid. Prophylactic therapy cannot be required by the employer. If a true exposure occurred, the entire group of potentially exposed workers should be observed for signs of active tuberculosis with greater vigilance.

In view of the complex medical and legal issues involved, screening for tuberculosis should be conducted by health care professionals and supervised by a physician trained in infectious diseases and/or occupational medicine. Early and frequent involvement of the local health department can confirm the appropriateness of the approach and deflect some of the distrust of management (see below).

COMMUNICATING TO EMPLOYEES

Although there is a body of literature that explores hazard communication in the setting of workplace exposure, the communications scenario more closely resembles a community-based exposure.[7] In workplaces in which exposures can be anticipated, there is mandated education and, often, personal protective equipment. An exposure is experienced as a personal event. In contrast, the unforeseen workplace exposure tends to involve a larger number of people and binds them together in a common experience. In addition, a number of issues quite specific to infection control are raised.

Typically, exposure to tuberculosis is unexpected and workers have varying degrees of knowledge and concern. The challenge of communicating information that would help workers to accurately assess their risk in this setting is great. The anxiety engendered by the initial rumors and announcements may prevent appropriate learning.

In some instances, such as in case 2, the magnitude of employees' concerns far exceeds the circumstances. The cluster of positive PPDs was "created" by a compulsive physician's assistant, new to the community, who was routinely testing a previously unscreened population of adults in their 50s for tuberculosis. The large employee demand for screening was driven by several other factors: persistent concerns about air quality and temperature, recent local reports of resistant tuberculosis, and a general distrust of management due to impending layoffs. Employees' anxieties were fueled by informal communications (rumors) and a vociferous resistance by a few angry workers to reasonable discussion. Although it was clear to management that no useful information would emerge from additional screening, a decision to conduct an on-site voluntary screening program was made. This appeared to be the only method to ensure that all employees' concerns were addressed. In addition, a screening program for people who are most fearful might provide an opportunity for individual counseling.

By contrast, the customer service employees discussed in case 3 were not especially anxious about the situation. It was their management that was concerned. In this instance, communications to the employees was limited to a simple memo recounting the circumstances and clearly stating that no exposure had occurred. Employees were invited to have their physicians call the medical director if there were any questions. The managers were asked to assist in the development of the memo so that all of the managers' concerns might be addressed.

In the one scenario in which there was a real risk to workers (case 1), the response was quite orderly. A meeting with all of the mailroom employees was held. A description of the initial exposure and plans for screening were distributed. All of the employees complied with the screening, and those found to have positive skin reactions were referred to their private physicians. All of these individuals complied with the investigators' request that they report back the results of the consultation with their own doctors.

The essential element of communication in this setting is to take control of the flow of information at the earliest possible juncture. This is best accomplished in small group meetings with the affected workers. Memoranda and general articles on tuberculosis will not be read carefully and are therefore no substitute for an open meeting. Any memos explaining the situation should be presented and discussed by a credible expert on infectious disease or occupational medicine. A plan for evaluation and follow-up of exposed individuals must be presented at this time. Employees must be given an opportunity to ask questions and ventilate their concerns.

A few caveats should be considered when preparing for a meeting to present information on exposures in the workplace. Management must be candid with the speaker in presenting the broad range of concerns that may motivate resistance to effective communication. Some thought must be given to the size of the group receiving the message—too small and some concerns will be unvoiced and not addressed—too large and the discussion can easily get out of hand. Managers should be present; they also may be exposed.

The tuberculosis screening process provides an opportunity for individual counseling on the risk of acquiring tuberculosis as well as detailed discussion of other issues raised by the exposure, such as HIV testing. The inadequacy of written communications alone to adequately address workers' concerns becomes very clear in the setting of individual counseling.

Results of the workplace screening should be made available to all concerned as soon as they are available. Again, a meeting may be helpful in bringing the matter to a close. It is essential to provide employees with an accurate written assessment of their exposure risk and the results of their screening. Giving employees a memo to take to their physicians will give credence to the trustworthiness of the investigation.

In presenting the clinical circumstances surrounding the exposure, one must be sensitive to the privacy of the source patient. A meeting to discuss the communications strategy with this employee is essential. The official story and what the employee will tell his/her coworkers must coincide. Although the identity of the source probably will be apparent to all, corporate communications should not specifically name the person. The clinical information provided to others should be the minimum required to allow outside physicians to make an appropriate assessment.

If a worker had been excluded from the workplace because of active tuberculosis, specific efforts to welcome him or her on returning are appropriate. Not infrequently, the source patient may be HIV-positive. In spite of the best efforts of medical personnel and human resources to maintain privacy and confidentiality of this information, other employees are likely to suspect or know. In some situations, additional education and counseling regarding HIV transmission may be warranted. Whether the diagnosis is tuberculosis, AIDS, or both, such individuals are protected under the Americans with Disabilities Act, and inappropriate exclusion from the workplace or other differential treatment may subject the employer to legal action.

The most effective communications strategy begins before any incident occurs. Middle level managers must be aware of appropriate policies and procedures and educated in their application. They also must know how to initiate the involvement of medical resources and be ready to participate in efforts to collect information and communicate with the employees.

CONCLUSIONS

A significant number of workplace exposures can be prevented or minimized by an appropriate level of vigilance. Policies and procedures that require evaluation of workers suspected of having active tuberculosis are essential for all workplaces.

An investigation conducted by medical personnel with expertise in infectious diseases and/or occupational medicine can minimize further exposure to tuberculosis and lay the foundation for an effective communications strategy.

The management of employees' anxieties and concerns depends on use of as many means as possible to reach workers; individual counseling, small group meetings, and written materials are a good beginning. Communications efforts should be reinforced by enlisting the employees' own physicians and local health agencies.

There are two goals to keep in mind in a workplace tuberculosis exposure. The first is to identify, evaluate, and treat any worker that has been exposed. The second is to ensure that all workers' concerns are addressed. The two are not always identical; sometimes it may be necessary to take extra steps, such as a voluntary screening, to help bring an investigation to a close. Although workplace outbreaks of tuberculosis are not likely, meticulous attention to reasonable principles of investigation, evaluation, and communication can minimize the impact of any occurrences.

REFERENCES

1. Centers for Disease Control: A strategic plan for the elimination of tuberculosis in the United States. MMWR 38(S-3):1–25, 1989.
2. Centers for Disease Control and Prevention: Draft guidelines for preventing the transmission of tuberculosis in health care facilities, 2nd ed; Notice of comment period. Federal Register 58:52810–52853, October 12, 1993.
3. Centers for Disease Control and Prevention: Tuberculosis control laws—United States, 1993. MMWR 42(RR-15):16, 1993.
4. Gottridge J, et al: The non-utility of chest roentgenography in asymptomatic patients with positive tuberculin test result. Arch Intern Med 149:1660–1664, 1989.
5. New York Times: California school becomes notorious for epidemic of TB. Page A1, July 18, 1994.
6. Snider DE Jr: Bacille Calmette-Guérin vaccinations and tuberculin skin test. JAMA 253:3438–3439, 1985.
7. Viscusi WK, Magat WA: Learning About Risk: Consumer and Worker Responses to Hazard Information. Cambridge, MA, Harvard University Press, 1987.

Statement of Ownership, Management and Circulation
(Required by Section 3685, Title 39, United States Code)

1A. Title of publication: OCCUPATIONAL MEDICINE: State of the Art Reviews
1B. Publication number: 0885114X
2. Date of filing: September 30, 1994
3. Frequency of issue: Quarterly
3A. Number of issues published annually: 4
3B. Annual subscription price: $82.00
4. Complete mailing address of known office of publication: 210 South 13th St., Philadelphia, PA 19107
5. Complete mailing address of the headquarters of general business of the publisher: 210 South 13th St., Philadelphia, PA 19107
6. Full names and complete mailing addresses of publisher, editor, and managing editor:
Publisher: HANLEY & BELFUS, INC., 210 S. 13th St., Philadelphia, PA 19107
Editor: Virginia B. Baskerville, HANLEY & BELFUS, INC., 210 S. 13th St., Philadelphia, PA 19107
Managing editor: Virginia B. Baskerville, HANLEY & BELFUS, INC., 210 S. 13th St., Philadelphia, PA 19107
7. Owner: HANLEY & BELFUS, INC., 210 S. 13th St., Philadelphia, PA 19107
Linda C. Belfus, 210 S. 13th St., Philadelphia, PA 19107
Holtzbrinck Publishing Holdings Limited Partnership, 415 Madison Ave., New York, NY 10017
8. Known bondholders, mortgagees, and other security holders owning or holding 1 percent or more of total amount of bonds, mortgages or other securities: None
9. Special rates: N.A.
10. Extent of nature of circulation:

	Average no. of copies ea. issue during prececing 12 months	Actual no. copies of single issues published nearest to filing date
A. Total no. copies (net press run)	2600	2660
B. Paid circulation:		
1. Sales through dealers, carriers, street vendors, and counter sales		
2. Mail subscription	1382	1382
C. Total paid and/or requested circulation	1382	1382
D. Free distribution by mail, carrier or other means samples, complimentary, and other free copies	6	6
E. Total distribution	1388	1388
F. Copies not distributed		
1. Office use, left over, unaccounted, spoiled after printing	1212	1272
2. Return from news agents	—	—
G. Total	2600	2660

11. I certify that the statements made by me above are correct and complete.

Virginia B. Baskerville, Editor

INDEX

Entries in **boldface** type indicate complete articles.